THE Bellamy HERBAL

Professor David Bellamy, botanist, writer and broadcaster has become one of the best-known and respected personalities in Britain. He is the author of 80 scientific papers and 34 books, many of which are bestselling children's titles. He has written and presented numerous television programmes both for the BBC and for independents. His programmes have won many national awards, including the Richard Dimbleby Award at BAFTA. He is president, patron or trustee of numerous conservation and environmental organisations and founded the Conservation Foundation in 1982. His autobiography, *Jolly Green Giant*, is also published by Century.

D0300232

ALSO BY DAVID BELLAMY

Bellamy on Botany (1972)
Bellamy's Britain (1974)
Green Worlds (1975)
It's Life (1976)
Botanic Action (1978)
Half of Paradise (1978)
Bellamy's Backyard Safari (1981)
Il Libro Verde (1981)
The Mouse Book (1983)
The Queen's Hidden Garden (1984)
Bellamy's Ireland (1986)
Bellamy's Changing Countryside (1987)
England's lost Wilderness (1990)
How Green Are You? (1991)
World Medicine: Plants Patients and People (1992),

Peatlands (1973)
Life Giving Sea (1975)
The World of Plants (1975)
Bellamy's Europe (1976)
Botanic Man (1978)
Forces of Life (1979)
The Great Seasons (1981)
Discovering the Countryside (1982,1983)
Bellamy's New World (1983)
I Spy (1985)
Turning the Tide (1986)
England's Last Wilderness (1989)
Wilderness Britain (1990)
Tomorrow's Earth (1991)
Blooming Bellamy (1993)
Trees of the World (1993)

and

Jolly Green Giant (2002)

THE Bellamy HERBAL

*A Whole World Herbal Handbook
for 21st Century Families*

DAVID BELLAMY

BSc. PhD. Hon DSc, DUniv, FLS. OBE

C

CENTURY

Published by Century in 2003

3 5 7 9 10 8 6 4 2

Copyright © David Bellamy 2003

First published in the United Kingdom in 2003 by Century
The Random House Group Limited
20 Vauxhall Bridge Road, London, SW1V 2SA

Random House Australia (Pty) Limited
20 Alfred Street, Milsons Point, Sydney,
New South Wales 2061, Australia

Random House New Zealand Limited
18 Poland Road, Glenfield
Auckland 10, New Zealand

Random House South Africa (Pty) Limited
Endulini, 5a Jubilee Road, Parktown 2193, South Africa

The Random House Group Limited Reg. No. 954009

www.randomhouse.co.uk

A CIP catalogue record for this book
is available from the British Library

Papers used by Random House UK are
natural, recyclable products made from wood grown in
sustainable forests. The manufacturing processes conform to
the environmental regulations of the country of origin

ISBN 07126 83690

Designed by Peter Ward
Printed and bound in Great Britain by
Mackays of Chatham Ltd, Chatham, Kent

NOTE FROM THE PUBLISHER:

Any information given in this book is not intended to be taken as a replacement for medical advice. Any person with a condition requiring medical attention should consult a qualified medical practitioner or suitable therapist.

The publisher and author are not responsible for any goods and/or services offered or referred to in this book and expressly disclaim all liability in connection with the fulfillment of orders for any such goods and/or services and for any damage, loss or expense to the person or property arising out of or relating to them.

To Thomas James Bellamy, MPS and Theo Bellamy,
his great grandson. I wish they had met.

Acknowledgements

Helen Knowles CSCT Dip, ITEC, E-C Therapy Practitioner, BRCP and ICM advisor to the Silver Crystal Research Project, and advisor to ICM for Aromatherapeutic oils, for keeping me completely up to date with developments in Herbal medicine. My thanks are also due to Rufus Bellamy for computer advice and guidance.

For further information please see
www.herbsphere.org

Contents

Fuel for Thought in the Game of Life

When you buy that next family car, be it saloon, hatchback, sports or macho four-wheel drive, you will make sure you know that all the important bits work and when it will have to be fuelled and serviced to keep it in running order. You'll read the instruction manual and follow the instructions. If you don't, the cost of keeping it on the road will escalate and the life of your car will be limited. It's also true that the more sophisticated the model, the more need there is to have it serviced by an expert.

Of course, you want to get it on the road and take it for a spin, so first things first. Which is the right fuel – diesel or petrol? the right octane rating? lead-free? plus a squirt of upper-cylinder lubrication? Get that right and off you go, a satisfied customer and a satisfied car until the next service station or service, when the oil will be changed, fluid levels and brakes checked, engine and transmission tuned, wheels and tyres balanced and reflated and, if necessary, bits and pieces replaced. Needless to say, an accident, serious or minor, may relegate it to the body shop, repair bay or scrap heap.

The same should be true of your body, the only difference being that as you can't go out and buy a new one, you have got to make it last for life. So reading the instruction manual and following the rules are of vital importance. Read all about it and if anything goes wrong, always seek expert advice.

The prototype human being was under development in Africa around five million years ago. Its design is thanks to Creative Evolution plc, a family business that had been hard at work since the year 3,600,000,000 BP (Before Present). Eve and Adam, the local dealers in the Rift Valley of Africa, unveiled the first top-of-the-range model some 500,000 BP. Today it comes in a variety of shapes, trims, customs and colours that all go under the trade name of *Homo sapiens*.

It's a basic model that has taken over the world marketplace, to the extent that today there are more people on the road of life than have ever lived before – over six billion of us.

If you are tempted to ask how herbs and herbal health can be the subject of a book now that humanity is dipping sixty billion toes in the hi-tech waters of the twenty-first century, all we need to do is go back to the basic question of fuel.

With all living things, fuel not only keeps them going but contains everything to keep them serviced and in repair. But put the wrong fuel in the tank, and you've got real problems. It's true to say that the basic model human being has been fuelled and serviced in the same way for 99.99+ per cent of its existence: plants and animals gathered from the wild have been washed down with water from springs, streams, lakes and rivers. In other words, the energy and raw materials that fuelled the success of our immediate ancestors for almost five million years were unprocessed plants and animals, the type and proportion consumed depending on where they lived. Organic wholefood provided everything to keep the human race going, growing, serviced and on the road to success – everything, including the twenty-five chemical elements of which we are made, not least those all-important trace elements that we hear so much about.

TRACE ELEMENTS

copper This is the same stuff that was in wireless sets when they contained wires. Copper is vital to the development and maintenance of the heart and the blood system, the structure and functioning of the central nervous system (brain and spinal cord), the integrity of the skeleton and even the health of your hair. Stop-press research reveals that skin patches that deliver high doses of copper to the bloodstream can reduce both the inflammation and the pain of arthritis.

magnesium This strange metal, used as flash powder by early photographers, plays an important role in every one of the cells that make up our bodies in the manufacture of proteins, the transfer of energy and the contraction of muscles. It is also the key constituent of chlorophyll in green plants, without which there would be a very different sort of life on earth.

zinc Used for galvanising pipes, zinc also galvanises us into action, for it is absolutely necessary for the normal cell division which allows us to grow, keeps our bodies in repair and replaces the two million red blood corpuscles that age and die every second. It also plays important roles in the normal functions of all these cells. The key role of this mineral, which is poisonous in too large doses, was discovered only in 1963 during a study of the health of boys living in the Nile delta. They all suffered from growth retardation, late development of sexual maturity and enlargement of internal organs, coupled with a strange desire to eat clay – the clay contained zinc. All symptoms were found to be curable by the addition of zinc to their diets. Today in the developed world, the lack of sufficient dietary zinc is linked to hyperactivity and its related syndromes in children.

manganese Used in high-performance alloys, a minute amount (10–20 milligrams – 0.0000006 per cent of your body weight) is of key importance in the formation of mucopolysaccharides, without which your bones, cartilages and ligaments – in fact the whole you – would fall to pieces.

molybdenum Only 9mg of this strange mineral is found in your body, yet without it biochemical reactions important in the working of all your cells could not get going.

selenium Now helping British Petroleum and other groups concerned to convert solar power into electricity in solar arrays, selenium has for millions of years helped living cells store energy and order the processes of life. Key in the manufacture of lipids, active components of cell membranes which help order our living chemistry, selenium aids the clotting of blood, is beneficial to our immune systems and, until AIDS poked its disruptive head on to the scene, helped protect our bodies from bacterial and viral attack.

It has been thought since the 1960s that selenium supplements might prevent dietary-linked cancers, and as I write this piece the medical fraternity is setting up a huge international trial designed to find out if selenium can reduce the incidence of lung, bowel and prostate cancers. Fifty-two thousand people from the USA and six European countries, including nine thousand from Britain, are being recruited to test the theory. Volunteers aged between sixty and seventy-four will take either a pill containing selenium or an inactive (placebo) pill for five years, but they will not know which they have been taking until the end of the trial. The researchers hope that couples will remind each other to take their pills. Other advice is also given, such as that selenium and vitamin C supplements should not be taken together.

The importance of these trace elements is clear. For example, certain parts of Western Australia have some of the oldest soils in the world, so old that much of the goodness of the trace elements has long since disappeared; in fact, they are so poor in minerals that in order to raise a crop of winter wheat, let alone the sheep that feed on the stubble, the farmers have to use special fertilisers containing – yes, molybdenum, zinc, copper and manganese.

Why, you may ask, should all these essential goodies be stored away in odd parts of plants and animals ready for our use? The answer is to do with the fact that we are what we eat. Plants get trace elements from the soil, animals get theirs from the plants they eat and the water they drink, so we get ours at second or third hand. The fact is that, just like you and me, plants are made of millions of living cells which, at the level of their living chemistry, are in many respects very much like ours. Plants are made of simple elements, of exactly the same building-blocks as we are: carbohydrates, fats and proteins – organic (that is, natural, life-synthesised) chemicals that are also, in the main, exactly the same as ours.

Primitive bacteria pioneered the chemical processes of life at least three billion years before there were any plants or animals. And they needed trace elements just as much as we and all plants and animals do. This is why we don't need to eat clay or soil: the plants have already harvested the elements for us, presenting them in flavoursome recyclable packets that come complete with the energy we need, all ready to do us good.

Homo sapiens is indeed one of the current winners in a universal game called Mineral, Vegetable and Animal, a game of survival that has been played on our planet for at least thirty-six thousand millennia. The only problem is that we are now showing signs of beginning to take on the role of the weakest link. Perhaps it's time to review the basic players in the game of chemical Lego.

ELEMENTS

The universe of which we are a product and hence a part is made up of 115 basic building-blocks called elements. Some of these, like mercury, lead and oxygen, are deadly poisonous, so it is fortunate that the living chemistry has had a long time to come to terms with its elemental environment. Throughout evolutionary time the living system has armed itself against environmental problems deriving from the elemental level upward, aiming for immunity and beyond, to the extent that only twenty-five elements have become part of life's rich chemistry. Most of these appear in about the same proportion in all living things, and the rest have been relegated to a mere backround role, part of the environment.

A catalogue of those elements that make you and me can be found below, together with their proportions (given in descending order) in the average (70-kilogram) adult human body plus a little information to whet your appetite (which is itself a chemical reaction).

oxygen Making up 61% of the mass of your body, this highly corrosive gas is not only the most abundant element in you but also the third most abundant in the universe. Fortunately, most of it is locked away safe in H_2O, the water that makes up around 80% of you.

carbon (23%) One of the most common elements being given out by dying stars into the interstellar void, and a main structural component of the living chemistry, forming the backbone chemicals of the carbohydrates, fats and proteins of cosmic you.

hydrogen (10%) The first element of creation and still the most abundant in the universe. Most of this explosive gas is locked up safe in your water but some, forming hydrogen bonds, is used to shape your working chemicals.

nitrogen (2.6%) An inert gas that makes up 78% of the air you breathe and is a key component of your working chemistry and of fertilisers.

calcium (1.4%) Although poisonous, this is the most abundant metal in our bodies, and is stored away safely in bones and teeth. It also helps intracellular membranes work properly, aids muscle contraction, nerve impulses, blood clotting and chemistry, and cell division, as well as triggering hormone release.

phosphorus (1.1%) Although in excess it is a deadly poison, without this element the energy contained in your food could not be put to work in your body. Our bodies produce, use and recycle 1 kilogram of adenosine triphosphate every hour – that's why it is another important component of fertilisers. Adenosine triphosphate is a key body chemical in the use of energy, and phosphorus is required to make it.

sulphur (0.2%) Thank goodness sulphur is produced by volcanic action, because there is no major cycle that returns sulphur back on to land once it has been washed down into the sea. Without sufficient sulphur all living things would collapse, for down at the level of cellular chemistry special bonds that contain sulphur keep our proteins in good shape.

potassium (0.2%) A chemical key to many crucially important living processes. We have more potassium than sodium in our blood and in our bodies generally. It is thought that this balance reflects the composition of the Precambrian seas before life became complex enough to begin to take over the land around 600 million years ago.

sodium (0.14%) Modern-day seawater contains more sodium than potassium, one reason why marine plants and animals use a lot of energy keeping the stuff out. However, enough must be allowed in for without salt life loses its savour and all sorts of problems much worse than cramp raise their painful heads.

chlorine (0.12%) Sodium plus chlorine make salt. Chlorine is a very toxic gas but when dissolved in water it is crucially important to key life processes. There is even evidence that the white blood corpuscles that defend our bodies may produce elemental chlorine to kill bacteria – real chemical warfare deep inside you.

From this point on, the amounts are so small that the proportion of your body made of the particular element will be shown in another way – not as a percentage of body mass but as the number of parts of that element in every million parts of your body weight, 'ppm' for short.

magnesium (270ppm) Without this flashy element chlorophyll would not be able to capture the energy of the sun – hence there would be no sugars and no oxygen in the atmosphere. On a more personal level it is of importance to our skeletons. Over a hundred of our enzymes would not work without it, our proteins would collapse and our genetic libraries would not replicate.

silicon (260ppm) Of great importance to our bones, connective tissues and skin, and in the form of silicon chips it is the basis of the IT revolution which is taking over our world. But watch it! The sad thing is that without silicon we would see the world through a glass darkly, for this very common element is important in the structure of our eyes.

iron (60ppm) Of crucial importance in transporting oxygen around our bodies, iron is the metal at the heart of haemoglobin, yet an intake of a mere 200mg per day can be toxic to adults.

fluorine (37ppm) Proven to be essential to the workings of our bodies, but too much in the wrong place can kill.

zinc (33ppm) Of key importance in more than 200 enzymes, zinc is also present in the complex proteins that are our genetic library. Too little zinc, like too tight underpants, may have an adverse effect on the production of sperm cells.

copper (1ppm) All living cells require copper to make them work. True blue-blooded animals like octopuses, snails and spiders use copper instead of iron to carry oxygen around their bodies.

manganese (0.2ppm) A key component of ten of our key enzymes; one of these, called superoxide dismutase, protects our bodies from the oxygen in free radicals, which attack and destroy bodily tissues at the cellular level (see p. 3).

tin (0.2ppm) Proof of the essential nature of this element is lacking, but there is some evidence that it is of importance.

iodine (0.2ppm) Needed for our normal growth and development, most of our iodine is found in the thyroid and other life-control centres. Like most good things, too much causes problems. Remember how a dab of iodine used to hurt – it may have killed bacteria but it also caused tissue damage. Fifty years on, another stinging secret is out: a Ministry of Defence experiment to seed rain clouds with iodine had catastrophic results for Lynmouth, on the Devon coast, in 1952.

nickel (0.1ppm) Linked with healthy growth, but some people are very allergic to this useful metal, which keeps the shine on stainless steel.

molybdenum (0.1ppm) Essential to all living things in minute quantities, for it is the key component of ten enzymes that make the living world go round.

vanadium (0.1ppm) We need it, and so do the microbes that fix nitrogen from the air and make it available to our food plants.

chromium (0.03ppm) Helps our bodies to make use of the energy in glucose, and is found in greatest abundance in the placenta. Mum always has known best.

cobalt (0.02 ppm) At the heart of vitamin B_{12}; lack of the right sort of cobalt causes pernicious anaemia.

selenium (0.01 ppm) Found to be an essential element only in 1975, it is a key part of the enzyme glutathione peroxidase which gets rid of peroxidases before they can form those oxygen-releasing free radicals that can cost us a lot, healthwise.

So there you have it – a list of the inorganic chemicals of great importance to you and your health.

EARLY LIFE

All the evidence we have tells us that around four billion years ago there was no life on earth. The cooling planet was made of minerals, themselves made up of ninety-two chemical elements which were in the process of stabilising to form the rocks of the surface crust and a primitive atmosphere. As soon as the temperature of the still young planet fell below 100°C, any depressions in the crust began to fill with water. The atmosphere was made of a mixture of toxic gases and vapours with no free oxygen at all. Not a very nice place in which to live, but as there was then no life on earth it didn't really matter.

The rocks of the earth's crust are mainly made of oxygen and silicon bound together as oxides of silicon, with sixteen other elements and traces of another eight. The others are usually found concentrated as ores in specific places. Then, around 3.6 billion years ago something fantastic happened (we are still arguing about exactly what, but all will no doubt be revealed in the fullness of time): living chemical structures, organic chemicals made mainly of only four elements – carbon, hydrogen, oxygen and nitrogen – began their long makeover of Mother Earth. Some people speak of creation, some of evolution, and for the sake of a quiet life I will use the term 'creative evolution'.

At first the chemistry or life was on the slow burner of anaerobic respiration, a fancy name for fermentation or composting – processes still at work today in the brewer's vat and deep in the compost heap, processes that released some of the energy available in the organic fuels made and used by the simple bacteria of those far-off times. The by-products included carbon dioxide, methane and water vapour, all greenhouse gases warming the primitive atmosphere, as well as alcohol and other energy-rich wastes. Actual burning, as we all know, is a more spectacular process releasing much more of the energy from the fuel in the form of heat and light, but it needs oxygen if it is going to happen.

For better or worse, a billion years later new forms of life developed that we now call photosynthetic bacteria and blue-green algae, not-so-simple microscopic organisms that had developed the ability to release oxygen from reactions with minerals, water and organic chemicals. With oxygen now free in the environment, fire became a possibility, as did aerobic respiration which would release much more of the energy contained in the organic fuels. But free oxygen brought problems wherever there were things that could be oxidised, especially down at the level of cell chemistry. Any free oxygen released within the cell could attack the living structures, in effect burning them up. In consequence a whole new armamentarium of fire-fighting chemicals that we now call 'antioxidants' had to be mustered to protect the cells from rogue free radicals. Antioxidants were probably not the first, but they are certainly among the most important, parts of life's immune system, protecting the core functions of living from attack by alien atoms, compounds or other living systems.

So it was that life began to shift on to the front burner of aerobic respiration, using up some of the oxygen and so helping to keep this potentially toxic gas in balance in the atmosphere. The frightening thing is that, today, if the level of free oxygen in the atmosphere increased by only 3 per cent, all the organic material on the face of the earth would go up in smoke. Fortunately, when all this was starting to happen the only organic chemicals were those produced by microscopic bacteria living in damp places, so there wasn't much to burn. It was going to take another three billion years to sort out the oxygen problem so that complex vegetables and animals could begin to play the game of life.

So minerals in the form of elements provide the raw materials for the growth of plants, which use the energy of the sun to make more of themselves – that is, all the sugars, proteins, fats and hormones they are made of. Animals eat plants or other animals, usually a mixture of both, and so for over three billion years the whole of the earth's food resource went from strength to strength – from bacteria to plants to animals and back via fungi and bacteria to the soil, the eternal biogeochemical cycle that is life as we now know it. With geological time on its hands natural selection was able to sort out the good from the bad; chemicals that poisoned a certain part of the living chemistry could in time become accepted, as they underwent subtle changes which augured well for their survival. The Russians have a novel term for these – 'adaptogens', living chemicals that can adapt to change and hence help the host system win in the survival stakes. Over time, immune systems as we are now beginning to understand them, were put in place. Systems so complex that, for instance, skin grafts even between identical twins face rejection.

MORE BASIC COMPONENTS

Carbohydrate is the correct term for sugars; all are made up of carbon, hydrogen and oxygen and all store energy originally fixed by plants. Some, like glucose, sucrose, lactose, fructose and mannose, are small moles that dissolve in water and so are always ready for action. Others, like starch and our own special energy store called 'glycogen', are large polymers that don't dissolve easily and so can store the energy out of harm's way until needed, when they are mobilised ready for use.

Fats, or *lipids*, are made of exactly the same three elements as the carbohydrates but they do not dissolve in water. Another important difference is that they have much less 'problem oxygen' in their make-up and so are more efficient at storing energy. Lipids come in long chains made of carbon (hence, e.g., long-chain fatty acids) and perform all sorts of important body functions. At the intracellular level they make highly complex membranes, which keep desirables in and undesirables out of living cells. On the macro scale they protect and insulate our bodies and can give us a curvaceous shape or cause unsightly lumps and bumps.

Lipids come in two types. The majority are solid or semi-solid, and as they come saturated with hydrogen they are called 'saturated fatty acids'. We get most of these from animals, in lard, milk, butter and cheese, and from coconut and palm oil. Recent research has shown that too much of these is not good either for our shape or our wellbeing. Even the now dreaded cholesterol comes in two forms, high-density lipoprotein (HDL) and low-density lipoprotein (LDL). The former, though a scavenger, is a goody, for it picks up fat and cholesterol from the tissues and transports them to the liver where they can be broken down. LDL is a baddy, for in excess it can get into the tissues, plastering itself on to the surface of blood vessels and causing atheroschlerosis.

A smaller group, best referred to as oils, we get mainly from the plants we eat and also from fish; they do not contain as much hydrogen in their make-up and so are more fluid. These are called 'unsaturated fatty acids' and come in two types, mono- and polyunsaturated. Of all the fatty acids our bodies need, only linoleic, arachidonic and linolenic must be obtained from our food; the rest we can make from sugar. However, always bear in mind that although a little of what you fancy may do you good, too much may upset the living balance especially of our cell membrances and hence of our health.

Over the period of writing this book much research has been carried out on a naturally occurring lipid called 'conjugated linoleic acid'. CLA came into the full glare of media attention when this component of red meat was found to help prevent cancer. Further research revealed its presence in milk, butter, processed cheese – in fact, in just about everything we were and still are being advised to cut out of our diet.

Cows and other ruminants have symbiotic micro-organisms living in their stomachs which help digest the tough plant food they eat, releasing among other things linoleic acid, part of which is turned into CLA – a fact that became even more newsworthy when further research showed CLA to be an efficient fat-buster. Roars of applause sounded from certain quarters, especially when they discovered that it works by enhancing the ability of cell membranes to open up and allow the absorption of fats and other nutrients rather than just dumping them in store in fat cells. All this corroborates the findings of over a decade of research by nutritional scientist Michael Zemel from the University of Tennessee, indicating that milk and dairy products decrease the risk of obesity because of their calcium content.

What was lost sight of in all this pro-dairy hype was that the amount of CLA found in meat and dairy produce is very small compared to the saturated fats they contain. Great to boast about in the press, maybe, but not much good to those struggling with cholesterol stress brought about by relying too much on a dairy-rich diet.

This is certainly not a new cause to be argued, at least amongst Caucasian stock, for Hippocrates the 'Father of Medicine' repeatedly warned against the use of too much milk. Indeed, he advocated a milk-free diet for dealing with all manner of ailments, from diarrhoea through aching joints, wheezing and skin complaints to enfeebled babies – good counsel even for the 30 per cent that have been weaned on to lactose over seven thousand years of animal farming. The other seven out of ten people across the world avoid the lactose in cow's milk for fear of a whole range of health problems. For us Caucasians it seems an awful shame that, with the help of people, cows turn grass into such a fantastic range of tasty things – butter, cheese, full-fat milk, cream and yoghurt – all of which tempt us to eat too much.

The fact that CLA, which is now being produced from sunflower oil, has been shown to promote rapid loss of fat and the growth of muscles indicates why it rapidly became a popular dietary supplement among body-builders. People on both sides of the argument are keeping a welfare eye on this incredible bulk. One complicating fact may be that a casual pinta gleaned straight from the udder (or a few stinging nettles gathered to use as a spring tonic) may not be quite the same as stapling on the stuff, or buying a synthetic product containing high concentrations of the active principle. And if the trend towards instant litigation continues the day may soon be upon us when all natural fruits, vegetables and spices will have to be labelled with a full list of their chemical contents, fighting for space with governmental health warnings.

Over a two-week period in the summer of 2002 two reports hit the headlines, both relating to major studies on the use of big players in the field of dietary supplements and healthcare. The first reported that popping vitamin pills does nothing to reduce the risk of heart attacks, strokes and cancer and ended with more than a suggestion that eating fresh fruit and veg might do you a lot more good. The following week, enraged customers of the larger variety were suing certain fast-food chains for not getting the message over by labelling their products as unhealthy. The second report, which got blanket coverage on 10 July, stated that the much lauded hormone replacement therapy increases the risk of breast cancer – thus pointing to the fact that organic food could be an important part of healthcare.

Our incredible hulk is made of water held together by large, complex organic chemicals called *proteins*. These are made of twenty-three building-blocks called amino acids – your very own AA running-repairers – which are themselves made of carbon, oxygen and hydrogen just like sugars and lipids, but spiced with the potential and the problems of nitrogen. Proteins are the stuff of our enzymes, hair, skin, connective tissues, muscles, nerves and even our chromosomes, which store all the information to keep us working and let us and our partners swell the ranks of *Homo sapiens*. Enzymes are very active organic catalysts that kick-start and lubricate all the chemical reactions of all living things, and although they are all organic chemicals a number of them cannot do their vital work in the absence of those metallic trace elements mentioned earlier.

Our bodies rely on over twenty different secret agents licensed to kill or cure, special notelets, or chemical messengers, that are all made of lipids. Produced in the endocrine glands, *hormones* are transmitted by the blood and act as messengers within the body, keeping it in balance and speeding it into action when the need arises. If the level of any of these gets out of kilter so too do the innermost workings of our bodies.

Vitamins are in the main made by plants and appear ready-packed for our convenience. Vitamin A (retinol) maintains the general health of all your living cells and is essential for vision. Vitamin B is a complex of at least ten chemicals, needed for the growth and maintenance of healthy tissues and organs; from digestion, through blood formation to the transmission of nerve impulses, vitamins of this complex play important roles. Vitamin C (ascorbic acid), also important in the maintenance of healthy tissues, helps many enzymes, especially those used in the digestion and rebuilding of proteins; vitamin C also increases resistance against infection and speeds the healing of wounds. Vitamin D (calciferol) enables our skeletons and teeth to do their work. Vitamin E (tocopherol) protects membranes, helping them to function. Vitamin K (polyquinone) is essential for the clotting of blood. A, D, E and K are fat-soluble and B and C are water-soluble, which is why they can be lost through cooking or processing.

Then there's a strange chemical called vitamin P, which is actually a group of substances called 'bioflavonoids', the first substances known to act as protectors of capillaries, 'the smallest blood vessels in our bodies'. Oranges are a rich source of bioflavonoids, which appear to work best when taken with vitamin C.

WE ARE WHAT WE EAT

As I said earlier, we are what we eat, as are sheep, cows, pigs, chickens and tuna, and we all depend on plants, for they are at the base of every food chain. Fortunately for us, plants come complete with all those metals and minerals and most of the vitamins, amino acids, lipids and carbohydrates we need and that our bodies cannot make for themselves. So as animals started enjoying an ever more varied diet they found nature's own organic supermarket packed with most of what they needed to keep their bodies growing, going and in good health. As they could obtain all the building-blocks they required from their diet, it was a waste of energy and space on their own cellular production lines to have to make them. So in the same way that the dodo, faced with no predators in Mauritius, lost its power of flight, the ability of animals to synthesise certain of these crucially important substances slowly disappeared. Add to this the fact that the essential building-blocks don't come on their own but as a complete package meal, with all the other chemicals that have made the living world go round for millions of years. Adding nothing, taking nothing away, Mother Nature has always provided pure, unadulterated, glorious, organic wholefood.

The problem is that if we process food in the wrong way much of this goodness can disappear in the factory or down the kitchen sink, or be rendered into such a form that our bodies cannot make use of it. If you don't believe me take a look at the back of your cornflakes packet, one of the earlier examples of processed food. Never mind the free offer, just look at the list of minerals, vitamins and other food supplements the manufacturer has *added* to your healthful dietary fibre. Unless your cornflakes are natural, wholefood or organic, you will find these things listed on most of the different brands' packets, so they must be important. Here's the selection gleaned from my breakfast-time pack and a list of some of their natural sources.

Vitamin B_6: found in wheatgerm and bran, brown rice and corn.

Vitamin B_5: found in wheatgerm and bran.

Vitamin B_1 (thiamine): found in wheatgerm and bran, brown rice and wholemeal and wheat flour.

Iron: found in oatmeal and bran flakes.

In these days of consumerism there are, of course, so-called luxury cereals bursting with all sorts of other additives. Some of these cereals are very low in fibre and some are so topped up with saturated fats and sugar that perhaps they should carry health warnings, for in the psyche of the public, remember, cereals are good for you.

Wheat, rice, oats and corn (in botanical language *Triticum aestivum, Oryza sativa, Avena sativa* and *Zea mays*) contain many of the things we need for a healthful diet. So why, you might ask, all the additives? The sad truth is that the modern fad of food-processing, preserving, canning, cooking – even boiling – can take most of those healthful things out. So unless they are replaced we could begin to suffer from all sorts of nasty deficiency diseases. That's what this book is all about. *Homo sapiens* needs to work in conjunction with the plants described here, which, if given a chance, will continue to serve us well in health and sickness, just as they served our ancestors for millions of years.

Our daily intake of body fuel should be somewhere between 2,000 and 4,000 kilocalories, depending on size and activity level. Our food must also provide us with all the raw materials needed to keep us active, in repair and healthy. Energy to keep all our systems up and running is supplied mainly in the form of carbohydrates which our bodies utilise in the form of sugars, but it's important we have the right sort. Refined white sugar may satisfy the cravings of the sweet-tooth brigade, but too much of it certainly won't do your teeth and general health much good. Brown unrefined sugar and honey appear to be a lot better – but again, everything in moderation. Fats are a great way of storing energy for later use, which is why camels have humps. (Sadly, *we* get them in the wrong places.) Body-building and repair use energy and also require a good supply of lipids, amino acids, vitamins, hormones and minerals. Some of them we can make from other things, some we can recycle, and some we have to import in our food on a day-to-day basis.

Until very recently, the chemical environment and hence the chemical content of the food we eat had changed but little since the time of Eve and Adam. However, in the last two hundred years and especially in the last fifty, all that has changed. Chemists have been busy engineering new chemicals, many designed to kill other living things – insect pests, bacteria, viruses, fungi, weeds, rats, mice, rabbits, starlings and, yes, even people. Some of these chemicals are let loose on purpose, others escape by accident. All taint the environment. Need I remind you of the problems of DDT, thalidomide, mad cow disease or the earlier warnings set out in graphic detail in Rachel Carson's book, *Silent Spring*? – predictions that have lately come true across much of Britain.

Unhappily, it is now a fact that DDT residues are found even in the fat of penguins living in the Antarctic. We can only wonder if it makes them feel poorly or renders them insect-proof. It certainly did pere-grine falcons no good, for they almost became extinct across large areas of the world before the massive use of DDT was banned. Today many of our other once much more common birds like song thrush-es, skylarks and even sparrows are becoming rarer, and at the time of writing we don't know exactly why.

We worry about atomic radiation – and so we should, for in the wrong place it can kill. Chernobyl was a tragedy, but at least it helped part of the world agree that atomic power is not the cheap, safe alter-native to the burning of fossil fuels that it was once cracked up to be. But how about all the other radiations – radio waves (short, medium, long), hi-fi waves, microwaves and those emanating from transmission lines? New ones seem to be added to our environment every decade, and the media are full of scare stories while at the same time using and advertising the gadgets that produce these waves of concern.

Heavy metal on at full blare can certainly damage your hearing, strobe lights can trigger fits, and might mobile telephones and their masts be more than an auditory and visual nuisance in public places? What are all these waves and rumours of waves doing to us at our innermost electronic level? For our living organic chemistry works by the subtle cascading of electrons inside and between the atoms that make up our organic molecules. One of the most inspiring lecturers of my student days was a professor by the name of Albert Szent Gyorgi. Despite the fact that he got a Nobel Prize for it, his work investigating the relationships between electrons and cancer never received either public funding, or a nod of approval from the scientific establishment. Were his ideas just too way-out for the 1950s, or were the powers-that-were worried that serious science might shoot the commercial hijack-ing of science in the foot?

Enough of that. The last thing a good instruction manual should do is depress the reader, so here are two good bits of news. The first is that despite all the worries concerning our modern lifestyle, we the people of the rich world are all living a lot longer than our ancestors – proof positive that life in the fast lane can't be doing us *too* much harm. However, certain health problems are real causes of increasing con-cern. Allergies, cancer, strokes, multiple sclerosis, Alzheimer's, osteo-porosis, anorexia and hyperactivity are becoming more commonplace. So-called superbugs that are immune to all known antibiotics are raising their ugly heads, and then there is the scourge of BSE and AIDS. All these are causing us lots of anxiety, which leads to stress, then – bingo! depression, and another lifestyle syndrome takes over. This is where my next good-news story comes in: thanks to a common or backyard weed called St John's wort (*Hypericum perforatum*), even depression can be tackled.

Depression is nothing new, for over the centuries extract of St John's wort has been used to treat anxiety, especially with relation to childbirth. Sadly, over time this, like so many other well-tried herbal prescriptions, fell into disrepute with the established pharmaceutical industry, which was perhaps too busy patenting new synthetic drugs. So the herb of St John was relegated to the tea-bag end of treatment. However, recent research is showing that simple extracts of this herb contain natural chemicals called 'hypericins', that in clinical trials produced significant improvement in anxiety symptoms in women after four to six weeks' treatment. The big drug houses were quick to react and soon extracts of this 'weed' were outselling its nearest synthetic rival Prozac by six to one. Why this rapid rise to fame in the twenty-first century? Could it be because it works and has acceptable side-effects? But more of that, and stress, later.

What this book attempts to do is let you find out more about the amazing living thing that is you, by opening a window on to an even more amazing relationship – that between plants and human health. As we take a tour around the body and examine some of its ailments, we will discover how humans have over long centuries of trial, error and experimentation chosen plants to help them not only feed themselves in a healthy way but also heal themselves when things go wrong. What is perhaps most amazing is how this process not only continues today, but is being backed up, verified and moved forward by modern science. Unfortunately, I can present only a snapshot of how people and plants work together, for all too often when preparing this book we found that research hasn't yet gone far enough. Again and again we uncovered reports which showed that a plant has definite active ingredients, but the trail ended there and no more research had been done. With the current increased interest in herbal medicines, more research is at last being kick-started and the true potential of plant-based medicines unlocked, put into the public domain and promoted for the good of all humankind.

As you read on you will find that precaution prevails – hence the warnings that some herbal medicines and dietary supplements should not be used with certain modern drugs. For the sake of readability research references have been omitted, but every research fact presented has been documented and is stored in a database.

Since this book is primarily about singing the praises of food medicine, food stuff that is a good source of natural medicines, nearly every chapter includes fact boxes containing good counsel and up-to-the-minute news about age-old herbal remedies, mainly food medicine that has been tried and tested throughout the centuries. The boxes allow you to dip into the history, and the futures, of these plants. To get you in the mood, take a look at the first one.

ST JOHN'S WORT
Hypericum perforatum
EUROPE

St John's wort is a herb with diverse benefits. Once known as *oleum hyperici*, oil extracted from the plant has been used medicinally since the time of the ancient Greeks. Named after St John the Baptist, the word *hypericum* (derived from the Greek) means 'health' or 'over an apparition', a reference to the belief that the herb was so obnoxious to evil spirits that a whiff of it would cause them to flee. Its red juice signals the presence of the healing agent hypericin and was taken as a mystical symbol of Christ's blood. Traditionally, *oleum hyperici* is made using a base of cold-pressed virgin olive oil. The extraction process requires one thousand hours of infusion in the hot sun to maximise the transfer of the active principles into the oil. Herbalists use the oil externally for problems such as light burns, scars and bruises, especially in conjunction with calming oils such as calendula (marigold) or with witch hazel. The herb is also used in homoeopathy for pain and inflammation caused by nerve damage.

Research has shown that St John's wort oil is a sedative and

---

antispasmodic. This is reflected in the herb's ancient use for hysteria and nervous complaints. Hypericin and related chemicals in the plant have been found to be anxiolytic (anxiety-reducing), sedative and anti-inflammatory, and St John's wort oil is used to help calm nerve pain, bringing relief to some of those suffering from rheumatism and arthritis. The oil softens and relaxes taut, painful areas; its influence penetrates deep into tissue around bones and relieves nerve pain such as that of sciatica and lumbago.

1

How We Got the Way We Are – or, Why We Do Like to Be Beside the Seaside

It's strange to think that if all children were taught the same sign language from birth, then there would be no language barrier and all the world could sign away, one hopes, in perfect harmony. The problem would of course be, whose sign language would be selected as the world's norm. Scientists came across this problem a long time ago. They could all recognise a daisy or a dog, but when it came to talking about them, language barriers caused problems. Thanks to a Swedish botanist called Carolus Linnaeus (1707–78), scientists ended up giving every living thing a two-part Latin name, or binomial. They chose Latin because at that point in history Latin was to all intents and purposes a dead language; no one spoke it, so no one could grumble about an unfair advantage. Thus daisies became *Bellis perennis*, dogs *Canis familiaris* and people *Homo sapiens*. However, I am going to stick my neck out and say that *Homo aquaticus* might be a better name, and I will tell you why.

If, as theory would persuade us, our ancestors swung down from the trees and developed our two-legged stance and large-capacity brain while hunting and gathering on the open plains of Africa, why are we all so fond of the sea? Sir Alistair Hardy, one of the world's greatest marine scientists, advanced an explanation way back in the Flower Power 1960s. Hardy reckoned that as our ancestors came down from the trees heavy not only with edible fruits and leaves but with other primates – apes, monkeys and their like – they found a large slice of unoccupied waterside real estate waiting for them. Habitats beside the sea, bordering estuaries and alongside lakes and rivers, all of which were overflowing with good food: oysters, mussels, winkles, whelks, crayfish, shrimps, prawns, crabs, lobsters, fish, birds, turtles and mammals such as seals that had already made the transition from land to sea. All good to eat, and most of them easy to hunt and gather; who could resist the temptation to take up residence?

Living by the water (warm tropical seas and estuaries, for starters) and with the biggest shellfish soon out of reach, swimming and diving would have become vital for survival – a new way of life, with the buoyant water accelerating the development of walking upright on two legs. Think about it. You swim on all fours, but when you come to land you quickly find your feet and take on the upright stance, which would eventually come in very useful. As many four-legged animals can run as fast or faster than Linford Christie, the only other explanation for our two-leggedness was that it enabled our ancestors to see their prey over the tall savannah grasses. Why, then, do all hunting people keep a low profile when stalking their prey? That explanation just doesn't make sense, so the plot thickens.

Homo aquaticus – impossible, you may still be saying. But another main group of animals had already made a similar transition: some sixty million years before small hippopotamus-like mammals, finding that same rich food source beside the sea, had galloped in. Finding in the sea all they required, they learned to swim, and with no need to lie down and go to bed, let alone hibernate, they in time gave rise to the whales and dolphins. These were aquatic mammals without equal, which soon began to rule five-sevenths of this planet that we call Earth.

Like us, whales and dolphins have large brains and a layer of subcutaneous fat, and have lost most of their hairy coat. Hair is not a good thermal insulator when wet. Fat and blubber can't get wet, and they help make you buoyant. Like baby dolphins, human babies are born with a lot of fat, and if put in water before they are six months old they swim with eyes wide open and in control of their breathing. There is also good evidence that giving birth under water is good for both the human mother and her baby, which moves from one watery environment through another into the dry air above. All the evidence goes to show that we are all born swimmers, our early landlocked upbringing simply allowing us to forget how to do it. What other land-living animal can swim the English Channel and back and do a breath-held dive to 53 metres, as pearl and sponge divers do? *Homo aquaticus* – the evidence is there if you think about it.

With little or no bodily hair for insulation, we sweat to keep cool (a total waste of precious water, especially if trying to make a living in dry tropical savannah). The only true savannah animals that keep cool by sweating are water buck and hippos and they, sensible things, spend the heat of the day in water. All the rest stay in the shade when the sun is up except, of course, mad dogs and English people – and they did this long before ozone holes were discovered.

One final fact: people – yes, even the British – are basically fish-eaters. To prove it, most prehistoric rubbish dumps, when excavated, are found to abound in shells and the bones of fish rather than of mammals. Even London's diet up until the start of the last century included lots of whelks, winkles, oysters, cockles and mussels 'alive, alive-oh' gathered from the Thames estuary. As if to prove it, 280 out of the 340 main-course dishes in Mrs Beeton's famous cookery book are of fish, and her breakfast menus also centre on fish.

Why should we have become so hooked on fish? Professor John Deakin suggests that our fish diet may have been the key that allowed the development of our large brains. He argues that shellfish and inshore fish provide us with a balanced source of those all-important omega-6 and omega-3 unsaturated fatty acids, the exact ones that in a 1 to 1 ratio make up the bulk of the brains of all mammals. He also points out that during pregnancy (when a large part of our brains is being put in place) the placenta selectively concentrates these raw materials in the blood that nurtures the developing embryo. Of all the large mammals, dolphins and humans have the largest brains in relation to their body size. This means ample computer space to do all the things they and we do so well: control and run complex bodies, communicate, lead social lives and educate ourselves and our families in the art of survival – survival for us and, we hope, for the living planet upon which we all depend. Read on, for this manual of herbal health-care is part of your survival kit.

We humans and our immediate ancestors have made use of fire for at least four hundred thousand years, and before that wildfire must have added tasty ready-cooked morsels to the diet. When it came to animals they usually killed them first, but creatures like oysters were eaten alive! Thank goodness we can't hear them scream – perhaps that's an important part of our immune systems.

Like us, all living things are made of little packets called 'cells'. If you took a living cell from a potato, an apple, a sheep and a chimpanzee, our closest relative, they would have an awful lot in common. Each is a bag full of living chemicals – sugars, fats and proteins, enzymes, vitamins, hormones – or as the trading paper the *Exchange and Mart* says, 'what have you', all working together to make that cell and its owner tick. Many of the basic metabolic systems are so similar that they are in effect interchangeable. That's why we have thrived for so long by eating other living things.

If any of you don't like the *Homo aquaticus* theory and want to stick with *Homo sapiens*, be my guest. Of course, you may be right, but even if you decide that your particular ancestors went the dry-land route they certainly would have been in need of water and so would have stuck close to rivers, lakes and streams, which also abounded in fish and shellfish. As we venture forth into the twenty-first century, fresh food of the right sort, including adequate amounts of fish, still makes very good sense.

More evidence is being uncovered all the time suggesting that the exploitation of marine food resources brought about an expansion in the range and complexity of human behaviour. Some even say that the importance of seafood in the diet of the Japanese may have played a part in their role as leaders in the electronic revolution. Sadly, over the past fifty years the intake of oily fish in Britain has fallen from 283 to 146 grams per week, despite the fact that for the last decade the powers that be have advised us to eat at least two 70g portions of oily fish. A recent study of more than 8,700 women found that premature deliveries fell from 7.1 per cent in women who ate no fish to 1.9 per cent in the group who had eaten even small amounts of fish at least once a week during the early months of pregnancy. Average birth weight and the length of pregnancy tended to increase, the more fish women ate. Fish such as canned tuna is not oily and does not do the job, but mackerel and sardines – even when canned – herring, salmon and trout are excellent sources of the complex of nutrients required. Those who dislike fish can always take a spoonful of cod liver oil for its mind-sharpening qualities, and for the squeamish there are fish-oil capsules.

It would probably be right to conclude that our ancestors ate any shellfish and invertebrates they could gather and any fish they could catch, and they probably did the same with the amphibians, reptiles, birds, mammals and even insects they encountered. We know that they soon learned the link between red tides and toxic mussel poisoning, for the first people who lived on the coast of California posted lookouts who would warn their people not to eat shellfish if the sea had turned red. We now know that the sea turns red on account of the abundance of plankton which produces toxins that make shellfish and even fish deadly poisonous to humans.

Another reason why the descendants of Eve may have liked to be beside the seaside was that many plants fringing our shorelines are edible and are always there, ready to be used in times of scarcity as 'famine foods'. Little wonder, then, that they were regarded in some awe as life-savers and so became part of herbal practice. The roots of sea beet and sea rocket were pounded and mixed with flour by the first people on both sides of the Atlantic. In China, the early-flowering 'scurvy Grass' was found by early seafarers, miraculously, to cure scurvy. We now know that scurvy – not so miraculously – is caused by a lack of vitamin C, and this cliff-hanging herb is full of it.

The leaves of sea lovage that used to grow in abundance on the cliffs and rocky shores of the UK were added to whey as a purgative for calves. Once used for uterine complaints, rheumatism and hysterical or neurotic disorders too, it is still a valued plant and used as a diuretic that also improves digestion and stimulates the circulation. Another seaside plant elevated from famine food to herbal fame is the sea onion. It contains scillarin, a chemical that stimulates the heart and is to this day cultivated for the drug industry in Egypt and Turkey. There is also the yellow horned Poppy, the root, stem, leaf and fruits of which are antibacterial. It grows in the most inhospitable of habitats, on coastal shingle banks in many parts of the world. Recently, in an effort to find alternative lighting from plant oils and waxes, the yellow horned poppy's oil has been investigated, and it is said to burn very cleanly in lamps. Now better known as a garden plant cultivar, prickly sea holly root continues to be used as a medicinal herb for certain urinary problems.

Many of these plants have been neglected over the past two to three thousand years, except by medicinal herbalists. The good news is that in our fast-moving modern world they are beginning to make a comeback, as wholefood additions to our shopping trolleys. At last, medical scientists and nutritionists are taking note of a whole wealth of food and herbal medicine waiting 'out there' beside the seaside, that age-old armamentarium of real healthfoods ready to meet the needs of our ailing modern age.

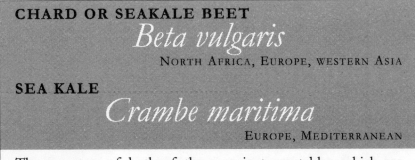

CHARD OR SEAKALE BEET
Beta vulgaris
NORTH AFRICA, EUROPE, WESTERN ASIA

SEA KALE
Crambe maritima
EUROPE, MEDITERRANEAN

The ancestors of both of these ancient vegetables, which are now coming back into fashion, were found in abundance growing along the coast where they provided a ready(slightly)-salted accompaniment to fish, shellfish and meat. Growing on shingle banks, they were often buried by storms; when excavated, then blanched, they were ready for eating, still with their full complement of vitamin C. Sea kale is much prized, especially in the Balearic Islands, where men with makeshift handcarts gather it for market. British ex-pats call it 'spinach sea kale' because, while the delicious tender white central rib eats like asparagus, the leaves cook down like spinach. It is definitely one vegetable that has gone up in the world, not least on account of its iron content and its ability to block free radicals in the fight against heart disease, cancer and strokes.

SEA BUCKTHORN
Hippophae rhamnoides
EUROPE, ASIA

This very spiny nitrogen-fixing shrub grows along the coasts and beside the alpine streams of Europe and Asia. Producing masses of orange berries, it is now being used extensively for landscaping. Used by both the Siberian peoples and the Tartars for food, drink *and* medicine, its freshly pressed juice can be taken against such ailments as the common cold, febrile conditions and exhaustion. The plant contains quantities of vitamins B_1, B_2, B_3, B_5, C, E and K, carotenes, fruit acids, flavones and antioxidant fatty oil, and its juice is widely used in the production of vitamin-rich medicaments and cosmetic preparations such as face-creams and toothpastes. In Tibet, it is used as a general panacea; its oil treats wounds and frostbite and digestive-mucus problems. A serotonin extract from the plant possesses anti-tumour properties, and the juice of the berries is used as a tonic against the common cold (appearing in healthfood stores as 'hippophae').

SEA HOLLY
Eryngium maritimum
EUROPE, MEDITERRANEAN

A sweet mucilaginous diuretic herb that is anti-inflammatory and an expectorant, eryngo has been used in medicine since at least the first century AD. The Greek physician Dioscorides advocated it as a cure for gaseous discomfort. The Latin name is thought to derive from the Greek word *eruggarein*, meaning 'to belch'. Its effectiveness has never officially been confirmed, yet anecdotally the root has been used with success for colds, coughs and bronchitis. It alleviates the pain of bladder and kidney-stones, kidney and urinary tract inflammation, urinating difficulties and oedema, and has even been used for skin disorders.

In England in the seventeenth century the herb was candied and enjoyed as a sweetmeat. Later, it was often made into a conserve and used to flavour jellies and toffee. Today it is employed internally for urinary infections, especially cystitis, urethritis and excessive urine production such as that experienced with diabetes and prostate complaints, and to treat enlargement or inflammation of the prostate gland.

SAMPHIRE
Crithmum maritimum
EUROPE, MEDITERRANEAN

From beyond recorded history, samphire has been gathered for salads, pickling and as an accompaniment to fish. Over three hundred years ago, the diarist John Evelyn remarked on 'its excellent Vertues and effects against the Spleen, cleansing the Passages, sharpening Appetite etc. so far preferable to most of our hotter Herbs'. Not to be confused with glasswort (of the *Salicornia* species), which grows between the tides, samphire is a succulent found among coastal rocks and cliffs. *Crithmum*, from the Greek, *krithe*, 'barley', refers to the ribbed ovate seeds. The common name 'samphire' comes from the French *sampière*, a shortening of 'herb of St Peter (the fisherman)'. Succulent samphire with its powerful salty taste is now making a comeback at fishmongers. It contains high levels of vitamin C and minerals, flavonoids, coumarins and gums. Recent research has also shown samphire's essential oils to be antioxidant and antimicrobial.

SEAWEEDS
Green, red and brown algae
WORLDWIDE

Plants by definition have roots, stems and leaves and the vast majority of them grow on land. Seaweeds have less differentiated single structures called 'thalli', and so are not true plants but must be called algae. Most grow on rocky shores around the world and come in three main colours – green, brown and red. As well as being a valuable source of food, seaweed has a wide range of medicinal uses. Kelp, for example, contains vitamin A and fucoxanthin, a carotenoid with anticarcinogenic properties. Its iodine content can help combat goitre, while an increase of iodine in the body increases thyroid-gland activity as well as the body's metabolic rate, and this can aid weight control. Detoxifying kelp contains alginates, molecules that have the unique property of being able to absorb heavy metals, radioactive substances and organic molecules such as cholesterol. The kelps are also used for arthritis treatment, to help cure sterility and for prostate trouble. Peruvians and Sherpas, on opposite sides of the world, carry little bags of kelp that they eat when at high altitudes, to aid breathing and restore tired leg muscles. The natural powder is also a good salt substitute.

The Japanese use seaweed as a food to counteract the effects of ageing, and it has been shown that cerebral haemorrhage and high blood pressure are rare in those who have a regular intake of these 'sea vegetables'. Seaweeds also have proven antibiotic properties, with different weeds working best on different bacteria. Recent research has shown that using alginate, which is bioresorbable, for the elongation of spinal-cord axons may in the future aid reconstructive surgery.

Given all these good properties, perhaps we should all try to add seaweeds to our diet. There is, however, one problem. All seaweeds accumulate toxic waste material including such nasty things as heavy metals and radioactive strontium, so the source of the raw material must be chosen with great care.

GARUM

Garum Armoricum

MEDITERRANEAN

We know that garum was being used by the neolithic occupants of north-western France and was further refined by the Celtic Druids. The liquor was originally described by Roman writer Pliny the Elder in his *Natural History* as consisting of the guts and flesh of fish and other parts that would otherwise be considered refuse, soaked in brine. The best garum was so highly valued that it brought fame not only to the people but to the nations that made it. Among those places famous for the quality of their garum was Pompeii, and in Rome's only surviving recipe book by one Apicius there are details of its use in a number of dishes.

Today it is used in the West and in Japan to tone up the nervous system and to conquer stress, fatigue, depression and anxiety. Innovative doctors in the USA are using this ancient remedy in place of the Federal Drug Administration's approved drugs Xanax, Prozac and Buspar.

2

How Did the World's Diets Get the Way They Are?

The much discussed 'human genome project', which first mapped all the genes that make us humans what we are, was completed as humanity took on the challenges of a new millennium. Thanks to this truly amazing bit of scientific research we know not only that, *having all descended from Adam and Eve, we are all close relatives*, but also that our truly amazing diversity depends on a mere thirty thousand genes. Most scientists thought we were going to be much more complex than this, with special genes coding all our potentials and problems. We now know that our genes code the production of 300,000 of those living Lego blocks called 'proteins'. As soon as each protein is formed within the cell it comes under the influence of the cellular environment, which is dependent in part on the food we eat and the water we drink, which are themselves at the mercy of the greater environment round about. The staggering thing is that the great diversity of people came about as the descendants of Eve and Adam took up the challenge of the various environments they encountered in their race across the world. As our ancestors moved into different climatic zones and environments, finding different foods and different challenges, natural selection produced the diversity of people we have today.

As the first people began to crowd into the best places beside the rivers and lakes of the Rift Valley, local food resources became depleted, so they either had to stay and fight for the food they required or move on in search of pastures new. The pushy 'hawks' probably stood their ground and the meek 'doves' probably turned the other cheek and moved on. On average, both groups had only a 50 per cent chance of survival. The few that had the ability to make a reasoned decision, and fight if they thought they would win or run if they thought they would lose, had on average a better chance in the survival stakes. They therefore won more often, and had a better chance to pass their genes on to another generation. They were the fittest in their particular round of what I like to call creative evolution by natural selection.

So they went forth and multiplied – north, south, east and west – on journeys of gastronomic discovery. No family saloons to speed them on their way and no service stations or shopping malls to provide for all their needs, they hunted and gathered what was available. They must have learned some of the tricks of the hunting-gathering trade while watching other animals. The maxim, 'if they can eat it, so can we', must have worked on many occasions, but sometimes it must have backfired. Take, for instance, the case of the yew tree (*Taxus baccata*). Twenty-four different sorts of British birds and animals can eat the leaves with no ill effects, but the same is not true for cows, horses and humans. So as they walked, these early people were on very steep learning curves. Given that there was no access to cold storage, a good gorge predated modern-day partying, and eating the gently rotting leftovers a few days later must have strengthened their gut flora and toned up their immune systems. They developed the most cosmopolitan of tastes, in essence eating everything that didn't make them ill and flavouring the bland and the bitter with what eventually came to be known as herbs and spices.

But it wasn't all plain sailing, for they encountered important groups of food plants harbouring what would be for them hidden dietary problems, like the legumes – peas, beans, pulses, grams and grains. The potential poisons that these vegetables contain range from complex substances that can kill to sugars such as raffinose and stachyose, which contain flatus-manufacturing substances. The problem is that our intestines do not contain the kind of enzymes that can break these substances down, and so as the bacteria do their best to clear the blockage they also produce lots of smelly gas. Fortunately for us, our ancestors learned by trial and error how to avoid such problem plants and, later, how to deal with the offending substances during the preparation of food, fermentation, soaking or cooking. Beware – today's countryside may abound with food for free, but a little bit of plant-identifying, or taxonomic, knowledge can go a long way to alleviate embarrassment or worse.

OUR FOOD HERITAGE

It is impossible to describe every nuance of world diet before the first agricultural revolution began to simplify it almost beyond recognition, because we have scant evidence on which to base any assumptions. All we can do is look at the plants and animals that have been handed down and that now figure in our diets, and surmise that at least some of them must have fuelled our immediate ancestors on their world travels.

To make the problem more bite-sized and digestible, we will group these foods into seven main geographical areas: (1) Africa; (2) the Mediterranean; (3) Europe and western Asia; (4) China, central and southern Asia; (5) the Pacific and South-East Asia; (6) the New World. And we can also break them down into the following six broad food types: (1) grains, cereals and the like; (2) roots and other underground storage organs; (3) vegetables (including salads, and stems) and some fruits; (4) soft, sweet fruits; (5) nuts; (6) herbs and spices; and for convenience we will add beverages (7) to the list. As with any form of classification there are overlaps between the types and the locations.

There should, of course, be a section allotted to fungi, for they are one of the most cosmopolitan of foods. Sadly, they are almost self-destructing and so leave few identifiable remains for us to find in excavations. For this reason we know little about their use in prehistoric times. So we will deal with fungi of which we have firmer evidence, as in the case of yeast, a microscopic harbinger of hangovers and flatulence. Without fungi, used across the millennia to put the rise into bread and dough into the pockets of bakers, brewers, distillers and excise men, world diets would be very different.

Most plants, and especially the staple whole-grain cereals, are rich in phytates, which have the unfortunate habit of binding minerals in the gut so that they cannot be taken up into our bloodstreams. Fortunately, the leavening of bread and other processes involving fermentation have solved this problem. Trehalose, the 'mushroom sugar', as its common name implies, is the main energy store of fungi. The fact that our digestive tract produces a specific enzyme that allows us to tap into this worldwide energy store shows that the friendly fungi have long been an important part of our diet. Certain fungi, though, can be far from friendly, as the name 'toadstool' – from the German words *Tod* ('death') and *Stuhl* ('stool') – so aptly reminds us. So have a care before venturing forth to collect your own. But it is not just the big showy fungi that cause problems: wheat and other cereals can get attacked by a fungus called 'ergot', which contains a deadly poison. Thank goodness its fruiting bodies are large enough to be recognised by the well informed eye.

There are, however, even smaller harbingers of death and destruction to be reckoned with. Food, especially nuts, stored badly can begin to rot, thanks to another group of not-so-fun guys called the moulds, some of which produce the dreaded aflatoxins, which can wreak havoc. Fortunately for us, many of these problems were encountered and solved, at least in part, by proper storage or adequate cooking or fermentation in the early days of agriculture.

In the light of modern research it is tempting to chart the travels of our ancestors by genetic differences that may well have come about as they faced the challenges of the different environments and foodstuffs they encountered on the way. These subtle differences would separate them into the following five groups: (1) sub-Saharan Africans; (2) Caucasians, including people from Europe, the Middle East and the Indian subcontinent; (3) Asians, including people from China, Japan, the Philippines and Siberia; (4) Pacific Islanders; and (5) Native Americans. Some would argue that such genetic differences should be taken into consideration when developing designer medicines. However, in this world of political correctness and given the escalating costs of pharmaceutical research, it is perhaps safer to stick with geographical regions. In the lists that follow some of the names are commonplace while others are so exotic that they won't yet be found in your dictionaries.

FOOD PLANTS STILL IN USE TODAY

1. Africa
   Grains finger millet, pearl millet, sorghum, teff
   Roots tiger nut, white Guinea yam, yellow Guinea yam
   Vegetables bambara groundnut, black-eyed pea, cow pea, gherkin, Hausa bean, melon, mongongo nut, morama bean, mubule, okra, palm heart, pigeon pea

Sweet fruits akee, banana, bottle gourd, carob, cashew apple, egusi melon, ensete banana, loofah, plantain, watermelon, wax gourd
Nuts palm-oil palm, sesame, yeheb
Herbs and spices caper, tamarind
Beverages coffee, kola nut, rooibos

2. The Mediterranean
Grains barley, hard wheat
Roots carrot, celeriac, chicory, leek, onion, radish, salsify, scorzonera
Vegetables broad bean, cabbage, cardoon, cauliflower, celery, cress, endive, fennel, garland chrysanthemum, globe artichoke, kale, lettuce, lentil, pea, radish, rocket, sea kale, shallot
Sweet fruits azarole, fig, clementine, date, grape, mulberry, olive, pomegranate, strawberry tree
Nuts almond, filbert, pine kernel, sweet chestnut, walnut
Herbs and spices bay laurel, coriander, cumin, garlic, lemon balm, marjoram, parsley, peppermint, rosemary, saffron, sage, summer savoury, winter savoury
Beverages aniseed (anise), juniper (gin), grape (wine), hops (beer), wormwood (absinthe)

3. Europe and western Asia
Grains barley, oats, rye, wheats
Roots beetroot, horseradish, kohlrabi, leek, onion, parsnip, radish, turnip, sugar beet, swede
Vegetables asparagus, aubergine, bistort, broccoli, Brussels sprout, cabbage, cardoon, cauliflower, celery, chard, chick pea, chicory, chives, fennel, Florentine fennel, kale, grass pea, horse gram, lovage, lablab pea, lentil, lettuce, orache, parsley, pot marigold, rape, samphire, sea kale, sorrel, Scottish lovage, scurvy grass, spinach, swede, turnip, watercress, white mustard, winter cress
Sweet fruits apple, bilberry, black mulberry, blackberry, blackcurrant, bramble, bullace, cherry (sour), cherry (sweet), cloudberry, cowberry, cranberry, date, damson, elderberry, gooseberry, greengage, grape, medlar, pear, plum, pomegranate, quince, raspberry, redcurrant, rowan, rose hip, service tree, sloe, strawberry, strawberry tree, white mulberry
Nuts hazelnut, pistachio, sweet chestnut, walnut

Herbs and spices angelica, basil, black mustard, chervil, caraway, coriander, dill, false horseradish, fenugreek, lemon grass, liquorice, mustard, origanum, peppermint, saffron, spearmint, tansy, tarragon, thyme, sweet cicely, white mustard

Beverages alecost (beer), chamomile (tea), hops (bitter beer), juniper (gin), southern wood (vermouth), wormwood (absinthe)

4. China, central and southern Asia

Grains buckwheat, millets (common, foxtail, little, Japanese), rice

Roots carrot, lesser yam, lotus

Vegetables bamboo shoots, beans (adzuki, cluster, lablab, Japanese), black gram, borassus palm, bunching onion, chick pea, chicory, Chinese water chestnut, cucumber, endive, garlic, green gram (mung bean), oilseed rape, onion, pigeon pea, pak-choi, pe-tsai, rape, red sorrel, rhubarb, soya bean, spinach, sugar palm, water chestnut, winged bean

Sweet fruits apricot, bitter gourd, cherry, citron, date, date plum, fig, kiwi fruit, kumquat, lemon, lime, loquat, longan, lychee, mango, nectarine, orange, peach, persimmon, Japanese plum, pomelo, rambutan, white mulberry, wineberry

Nuts ginkgo, gnetum, pistachio

Herbs and spices aniseed, basil, caper, cardamom, cinnamon, cassia, galangal, ginger, turmeric (allspice and black pepper)

Beverages cider apple, *fo ti tieng,* snakeroot, tea (China and Indian)

5. The Pacific and South-East Asia

Grains sago

Roots taro, greater yam

Vegetables New Zealand spinach, palm heart, sugar cane, winged bean

Sweet fruits banana, breadfruit, champedek, durian, grapefruit, jack fruit, mangosteen, marang, pomelo, star fruit

Nuts coconut, cycads, macadamia, Moreton Bay chestnut

Herbs and spices arrowroot, cinnamon, clove, mace, nutmeg

Beverages coconut (milk), kavakava (ceremonial/medicinal)

6. The New World

Grains and seeds grain amaranth, maize, quinoa, sunflower, wild rice

Roots buffalo gourd, cassava/manioc (tapioca), Jerusalem artichoke, mashua, new cocoyam, oca, potato, sweet potato, ulluco, yam, yam bean

Vegetables beans (broad, butter, horse, kidney, jack, scarlet runner, tepary), bell pepper, chayote, chicle, courgette, fig-leaf gourd, groundnut, marrow, pumpkin, squash, tomato, tamarillo

Sweet fruits abiu, New World apple, atemoya, avocado, bilberry, black sapota, blueberry, Cape gooseberry, ceriman, cherimoya, cowberry, cranberry, currants, custard apple (red and black), dragon fruit, dwarf Cape gooseberry, giant granadilla, gooseberry, guava, ilama, jaboticaba, mamey sapota, mountain pawpaw (papaya), passion fruit, pear, pineapple, plum, prickly pear, sapodilla, saw palmetto, soncoya, soursop, star apple, sweet sop, tomatillo, white sapota

Nuts black walnut, Brazil, butternut, cashew, monkey puzzle, pecan, pine kernel

Herbs and spices cayenne pepper, chilli, sugar maple, paprika, sweet honeyleaf, vanilla

Beverages Angostura (bitters), cacao (chocolate), guarana (tonic), quinine, sassafras (medicinal), slippery elm (medicinal), tequila (spirit), yerba maté (tonic)

For those of us living in the rich world many of these names will conjure up visual images, tastes and smells, whether of hard tack or of gourmet delights. Some of these images will be pleasant, some unpleasant. Some will be linked in our minds with words like 'bread' and 'chips' or commands like 'Eat up your greens.' In this world of supermarkets it has become difficult to imagine what it was like when your day was spent hunting and gathering the daily rations. How boring it must have been that what you ate was limited to what grew around your latest bit of real estate. But were those limitations really so great? Your family, or clan, ate everything their immediate ancestors had learned was edible – which amounted to an incredible range of textures and tastes even when eaten raw, and particularly with the added pleasures of caramelisation when the fire got too hot. In fact, the first fast food must have been the carcasses of animals collected ready-cooked after wildfire had passed that way – later turned into a technique of landscape management and perfected as 'fire-stick farming' by the Aboriginal people of Australia. And we can only guess how many favourite local foodstuffs were harvested to extinction. What did mammoth, giant sloth or giant elk taste like, let alone some of the plants they fed on? The above lists, which are not exhaustive, contain the survivors from what the then whole-earth herbal hyper-market had on offer.

The vast majority of today's fruits and vegetables are monsters compared to their wild ancestors, which the descendants of Eve learned to enjoy, select and finally domesticate, cultivate and farm. They would always have chosen the tastiest, the biggest and the best, those plants that would not be attacked by insects or diseases and those that would store well – thus sowing the seeds of plant and animal breeding and ultimately genetic modification. Perhaps it is us who are limited, for the staple components of the Western diet are a mere twenty-two plants and three sorts of animals, bred for uniformity and for profit, not for diversity. Yet thanks to our forefathers and -mothers we can still savour the pampered descendants of some things derived from the natural cornucopia that fuelled and serviced the long march of humanity across Mother Earth.

MOVEMENT AND CHANGE

At first, life in the tropical and subtropical climes with their year-round abundance of roots, shoots, fruits and game must have been easy. But as around 100,000 years ago people moved into drier and cooler zones, especially those climates still in the grip of the most recent of the seventeen glacial epochs that had again and again rejuvenated many of the soils of the higher latitudes and altitudes, things became more difficult. Less varied and more stringently seasonal diets would have begun to order people's way of life. The last great ice ages of which our immediate ancestors were a part lowered the sea levels, thereby opening up more fertile land and convenient escape routes to pastures new. Land bridges formed from Britain to Europe, Europe to North America and Asia to Australasia, opening up new lands and land-scapes, with new plants and animals there for the taking.

As Marsupials moved north from Australia, the Aboriginal people went the other way, wreaking havoc on the megafauna, the giant kangaroos, wombats and penguins. Wherever people went they came into conflict with the balance of natural resources. As the big herbivores were hunted out of existence the ranker vegetation grew out of control, changing the face of the island continent and becoming the fire hazard it still is. The first 1,300 years AD were a time of great change in the American ways of life. Later, antelope, bison and mammoth, as well as Mongolian people, streamed into America south of what is now the Bering Straits, and eight thousand years later were heading for homes on the islands of Tierra del Fuego. The fact that no less than thirty-five genera of large mammals went to the wall along their route leaves no doubt that our ancestors were not vegetarians. What's more, the omnivory of our more recent ancestors played at least some part both in their success and in what has come to be known as 'the Pleistocene overkill'. This was a sustained, wanton act of destruction 30,000 years ago that included people on both sides of the Atlantic, who would drive herds of reindeer and bison over cliffs, eating what they could and leaving piles of unbutchered carcasses as evidence of their disregard for the conservation of resources. Some, like the early Vikings, made more use of both land- and sea-based supplies of food, while others like the Japanese and the Inuit stuck to their marine diet, the latter only colonising Alaska around the time that Christ walked the earth and reaching Greenland as late as AD 1300.

At about the same time at the other end of the world the Maori people, following the example of all earlier human travellers, were getting stuck into the megafauna of, in their case, New Zealand: the giant moa birds, to be exact, for this last large slab of land to be discovered and colonised had no ground-living mammals to satisfy people's hunger and their lust for the kill. A mere five hundred years later, all the moas were extinct, forcing the people to return to the cultivation of the yams and sweet potato that had provendered their voyages of discovery.

It would be nice to be able to excuse these people on the grounds that they needed meat to provide them with the instant energy they required to keep warm and so cope with the cooler, harsher climates of the periglacial regions. The truth, however, is that the meat they craved came from free-range game, which is lean and hence energy-poor by nature, devoid of the lashings of fat that were bred in much later for the obvious reason of commercial gain in the marketplace.

This was the time of the neolithic revolution that introduced agriculture and kick-started civilisations in isolated areas across the world, some separated by oceans at that time heading back to their pre-glacial levels, others separated by mountains, deserts and forests. It was during this most recent thirty-thousand-year period that the human diet underwent its most dramatic change, as the domestication of animals and the development of crops led to the destruction of ever more forest, wetlands and natural vegetation and the organic soil that went with them. Agriculture was here to stay and, as it took hold of an ever greater area of the earth, the ultra-varied diets of the first-footers became ever more uniform.

The thirteen hundred years since the time when the Inuit found their present home on the edge of the still frozen North was one of immense change in the American way of life. The rapidly moving first-footers had wreaked their worst on the big game of the New World. The ones who stopped over in the warmer, more favoured forest-covered areas, the savannahs and prairies, developed an amazing variety of civilisations. I say 'amazing' because that's what they were: the Incas, Aztecs, Anasazi, Hopwellians, the Hohokam, Mogollons and the dwellers of the Appalachian woodlands. All built great landscape artefacts, the best of which are today sites of world heritage protected by international treaty.

I will now revise my spelling of the word 'amaizing', because their success came to depend essentially on one crop: maize, corn-on-the-cob to you, and *Zea mays* to botanists. In a little over ten thousand years they and their ancestors had selected and bred a wild plant growing in the hills of Mexico to become their staple food from the mouth of the St Lawrence River in Canada to central Chile. Today it is the main cash crop of the USA (followed by tomatoes, another native of Mexico). Christopher Columbus first saw this *mahiz* being grown by the locals on the island we now call Cuba in 1492. Its only disadvantage is that it is very demanding on fertiliser, rapidly depleting the soil of nutrients. So the success of both the plant and the people depended on stewardship that would keep the soil in good condition.

This one plant species thus became the mainstay of an agriculture that included beans (which came complete with their own fertiliser factories – root nodules full of nitrogen-fixing bacteria), squash and sunflowers. Squash, storing the sporadic rain in these semi-desert regions, provided pure water, energy, vitamins and lots of fibre in every mouthful, while sunflower seeds were and still are rich in brain-building unsaturated fatty acids.

Despite all this development, something went radically wrong about AD 1200, when these people's highly developed urban ways of life disappeared, leaving the land in the perhaps more capable hands of no less than 287 principal tribes whom we now properly call 'America's first people' – each family hunting, gathering, fishing and many still planting corn, beans, squash and sunflowers; each tribe making the most of everything its particular bit of real estate had to offer. It was almost as if a wind of change called 'Civilisation' had blown that way, had held sway during thirteen centuries of destruction of the landscape's natural balance and then, for some reason still not completely understood, had passed away, leaving the real survivors, those descendants of the first-footers who perhaps found spiritual satisfaction in a simpler, rural way of life. In an evolutionary sense, they were at that time the fittest and so had inherited their part of the earth, although no longer in its whole and wholesome state.

The same was true of all the other civilisations that waxed and waned during these earth-shattering thirty thousand years. Over two thousand years before the birth of Christ an inscription on a tomb in Luxor proves that famine was stalking the land: 'All Upper Egypt is dying of hunger, to such a degree that everyone has come to eating his children'; and according to Nefertiti, some hundred years later, 'The river of Egypt [was] empty. The birds no longer [laid] their eggs in the swamps of the delta.'

Over a millennium later Plato in his *Crito* warned the Greeks, who were then desperately searching for new and fertile lands, of the relationship between broad-leaved forest and the fertility of landscapes. He described changes he had seen in his own lifetime and, remarkably, spelt out the relationship between river flow and deep-rooted trees: 'The soil benefited from an annual rainfall which did not run to waste off the bare earth as it does today, but was absorbed in large quantities and stored in retentive layers of clay.'

The Romans followed suit, one of their motives in wishing to conquer the then known world being to find new and fertile land, to compensate for soil erosion at home and provide for their aspirations and their people's needs. Recent excavations of two Roman quarries in the eastern desert of Egypt have revealed the diet of the slaves who worked there during the first four centuries AD. No less than fifty-five different food plants and twenty sources of animal protein have been identified. Staples included wheat, lentils, dates, onions, garlic, olives, coriander, donkey meat and wine, all of which must have been brought in from settlements in the Nile Valley, a week's journey away across the desert, and fish from the Red Sea. Not bad for starters, and these foods would have been spiced up with non-essentials such as artichokes, hazelnuts, walnuts, pine-nuts, pomegranates, almonds, grapes, figs, watermelon, melon, cucumber, and even black pepper imported all the way from India. However, most surprising of all is the abundance of fresh green vegetables: lettuce, mint, cress, leaf beet and lots of cabbage. The presence of seeds of all these 'do you good' vegetables in the excavated quarries showed not only that the Romans looked after their hard-working slaves but that the vegetables were grown fresh on the spot. And the abundance of cabbage is not unconnected with the Latin *crambe repietita*, meaning 'warmed-up cabbage', an old, old version of 'Eat up your greens' and worth a mention in view of modern-day diets, with many people eating fewer varieties and smaller quantities of fresh fruits and vegetables, as well as taking less exercise – a root cause of lifestyle syndromes such as obesity, heart attack, strokes, bowel and prostate cancer and even diabetes.

The Romans were in the end overtaken by the barbarian hordes, who added plundering to their herdsman skills. The fact is that our forefathers and -mothers used to be in the business of hunting, gathering or growing all the food that they and their families required. It was hard work that used up the so-called structural fat, keeping them lean and healthy. (Back in those days they also used the fat gleaned from their animals for tallow candles, to light up their night lives.) But as people began to live in villages and towns where they earned their living doing other jobs, they became more sedentary and further removed from the land on which their food was grown. So it became more important to be able to store all sorts of foodstuffs for transport and for future use. Salting, smoking, curing, pickling, canning, stabilisation, refrigeration and irradiation are all processes that our food now undergoes, and all of them can cause problems. For instance, too much salt can cause high blood pressure and increases the risk of heart disease and strokes, as well as being linked to osteoporosis and stomach cancer. Although it's never mentioned on the packet, many processed foods now contain lots of additional salt, to which people unknowingly become addicted. Smoke residues in cured and burnt food can provoke cancer; vinegar, being acid, can upset digestion; food in cans may have been bleached, blanched or boiled – all of which can destroy important vitamins and cause the loss of minerals; while the pros and cons of irradiation are still being argued about.

Granaries have to be rat-, mouse- and insect-proof, or else such pests are controlled by culling, often with the use of poisons. Fortunately, refrigerators no longer contain ozone-destroying CFCs (chlorofluorocarbons) but, if not properly maintained, they can still become breeding grounds and hide-aways for hardy bacteria. Even antibiotics have helped cause the rapid evolution of the superbugs that are now threatening public health. Problems, problems – all part of the food-processing chain; but also benefits, benefits – at least in certain aspects of lifestyle.

Empires have come and gone, cashing in on the resources of others in a series of land grabs. Defending themselves as best they could, those same peoples were then gazumped by empires new and are now being offered the dubious promise of a global economy in which the richest 350 people together have more money than the poorest three billion – that is, half the current world population.

The dust-bowls of America, the awesome actually of Rachel Carson's *Silent Spring*, rampaging bush fires and soil salinity, the groundnut, mad-cow and foot-and-mouth fiascos, all warn that things can go radically wrong. And the fact that one-third of the people now trying to make a living from the once whole earth are facing problems of malnutrition and dirty water is but a symptom of a worldwide malaise. More and more farmers in the richest parts of the world are going bankrupt, and water shortages plague the rich and poor alike as the fears of ozone holes and global warming threaten the viability of insurance and the stability of the stock markets. The Rio summit and Kyoto conferences, the wars and the rumours of unlikely peace treaties, all show that as yet we have not got it right, and the fall-out is of global consequence. With over six billion people now knocking seven bells out of the soil and all the other earth systems that used to keep the planet in good health, the time has surely come to mend our ways and start to put the whole earth and the life-giving sea back into some semblance of biodiverse working order.

There are other signs, perhaps of more relevance to our own personal egos, that all is not well with our modern fast-food diet. The following table is from the work of an American dentist, Weston A. Price, who took a sailing sabbatical back in the early 1930s, a grand tour during which he studied the teeth of people around the world comparing those who still enjoyed their indigenous diet and those who had switched to the Western way.

Percentages of teeth attacked by decay in different peoples	*primitive diet*	*modernised diet*
Swiss	4.6	29.8
Gaels [Scots and Irish]	1.2	30.0
Eskimos [Inuit]	0.09	13.0
Northern Indians	0.16	21.5
Seminole Indians	4.0	40.0
Melanesians	0.38	29.0
Polynesians	0.32	21.9
Africans	0.20	6.8
Australian Aborigines	0.00	70.9
New Zealand Maori	0.01	55.3
Malays	0.09	20.6
Coastal Peruvians	0.04	40.0+
High Andes Indians	0.00	40.0+
Amazon Jungle Indians	0.00	40.0+

If this doesn't make you gnash your dentures and start worrying, then read on. Fifty years later august bodies such as the World Health Organisation and the Food and Agriculture Organisation of the United Nations agreed that there is a nutritional link between diet and heart disease. Ten years later, even the surgeon-generals' report on health in the USA agreed with this finding. Since then there has been increasing concern that other diseases including arthritis, colon and breast cancer, multiple sclerosis and Alzheimer's disease may be part of the same pattern of change.

It's time to mend our ways, both on a personal and on a planetary level – each one of us must think globally and act locally. Most important of all, we must conserve all that still remains of the diversity of all the plants and animals that the descendants of Eve found when they took over the then whole earth. Please, think on these things as you read on and as you make up your mind to fuel your lifestyle on the plants that follow.

RICE

Oryza sativa

CHINA, INDIA

Rice constitutes the bulk of the diet of almost two-thirds of the world's population. In its raw brown format it provides a good supply of energy in the form of starch – that's the white stuff – which makes up the bulk of each grain. At the heart of the grain is the germ, much smaller but stuffed full of goodies: fats, proteins, phosphates and vitamins, including vitamin E, the one that helps regulate the functions of the sex glands. All this, laid down for the healthy germination and strong early growth of the next generation of rice plants, comes safely double-wrapped in the bran layer and then an outer wrapper made up of two tiny leaves. The bran is rich in glutens (simple proteins) and minerals including those all-important trace elements. Rice bran is highly antioxidant, and a recent review of phytonutrients from rice bran has shown promising disease-preventing and health-related benefits. Preventive and/or neutraceutical effects from bran compounds and products have been detected in the treatment of diseases including hyperlipidaemia, fatty liver, kidney-stones and heart disease. Little wonder that when polished rice – that is, rice deprived of its outer layers – was first introduced into the economics of colonial rule, deficiency diseases became rife.

Rice has been cultivated in India and China for four thousand years and was first mentioned in traditional Chinese medicine in the seventh century AD. Until about the end of the last world war, rice water was commonly used in the West to soothe stomach irritations. As a diuretic, rice grain is useful for urinary dysfunction and excessive lactation; rice sprouts are used for poor appetite, indigestion and abdominal problems such as bloating. In the

East, the rhizomes are used for the night sweats associated with pneumonia and tuberculosis. Recent research has also found clinical uses for rice, e.g. in the treatment of children with persistent diarrhoea and to provide a simple, safe and cost-effective intervention in the form of thickened barium feeds to alleviate swallowing dysfunction. Rice germ is thought to be of benefit in the prevention of colorectal cancers.

Mirin, sweet rice wine, is the base of the ritual medicinal tonic called *o-toso*, used to herald the Japanese New Year. Brown rice vinegar, known as 'Japan's liquid treasure', is also used medicinally. It is now believed that amino acids present in the vinegar are partly responsible for its good effects, counteracting lactic-acid build-up in the blood which can cause fatigue, irritability and sore muscles. According to Dr Yoshio Takono of Shizuoka University, the twenty-two amino acids and sixteen organic acids found in authentic rice vinegar used as a condiment help prevent the formation of toxic fat peroxides, which contribute to cholesterol formation on blood-vessel walls and to ageing.

WHEAT
Triticum aestivum
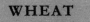
SOUTH-WEST ASIA

DURUM WHEAT
Triticum durum
SOUTH-WEST ASIA

BARLEY
Hordeum vulgare
SOUTH-WEST ASIA

Wheat is the basis of leavened bread, biscuits and cakes, while durum wheat makes pasta and noodles; together, the descendants of these grasses feed over two billion people across the world. And barley quenches their thirst and egos with beer and whisky. All three were discovered in the Fertile Crescent (which stretches from Armenia to Arabia), where the first farming communities were set up around ten thousand years ago. Like rice and all the other cereals in their natural unprocessed form, wheat provides us with endosperm, germ, bran and outer wrapper to keep us supplied with many of our basic bodily nutrients, as well as helping the body to function.

CORN-ON-THE-COB, MAIZE
Zea mays

NEW WORLD

When it comes to the serious stuff in cereals, corn is top of the pops in the Americas. Corn bread, flour, flakes, meal, tortillas – you name it, they eat it in one form or another. They even make a petrol called 'gasohol' from it – no wonder it's America's largest crop.

Native to Central America, maize has been cultivated for over seven thousand years in the New World. The plant tolerates a range of climates and can now be found growing all over the world. A cultural sacred plant of the Huichol Mexicans and the staple food of South America for over 5,500 years, it was used medically by the Aztecs in a maize-meal decoction to increase lactation. In folklore medicine, maize has been used for making poultices by Mayan, Incan and South American *curadores* (folk medicine exponents, or shamans) to treat bruises, swellings, sores and furunculae (boils). Fumigation by means of burning corn-cobs was employed by the Chickasaw peoples to treat the skin condition ichthyosis. An extract from the female flowers was used by the Aztecs and by the Chinese in the seventeenth century as a diuretic that lowers blood-sugar levels, stimulates bile flow and prevents the formation of kidney- and bladder-stones. Today, non-GM maize is not only a wholesome food but also a versatile medicinal plant which, being gluten-free, is especially useful for coeliac disease.

Research in China has shown that corn silk (the silky tuft at the tip of an ear of maize), known as *yu mi shu*, lowers blood pressure and shortens the blood-clotting period. The traditional use of corn silk as a tonic 'tea' and diuretic beneficial to the prostate and male reproductive organs requires further investigation. Corn silk's potassium content makes it a useful diuretic for many urinary ailments, especially prostate disorders. It soothes the irritation of the bladder and urethral walls caused by frequent urination. It is also reputed to have a helpful effect upon the kidneys, protecting against bladder- and kidney-stone formation and alleviating cystitis in women and enuresis in children. In China, maize has also been used to treat gallstones, hepatitis, jaundice, cirrhosis and oedema, and research indicates that it may help stimulate the flow of bile.

There is one down side: overindulgence in corn on or off the cob at one sitting can result in an upset stomach. The cellulose content is indigestible and too much at a time can cause painful flatulence. And there is another cloud on the cornfield horizon: some farm trials of corn that has been genetically modified to produce pharmaceuticals are already out of control and causing concern over contamination of other crops.

POTATO
Solanum tuberosum
New World

Gifts from the high mountain pastures of South America, potatoes are a fine source of nutrients. Richer in protein than even the fabled soya bean, a single tuber can supply an adult with half his or her daily need of vitamin C. They are also an outstanding source of potassium and a useful fount of vitamin B complex. Boiled or baked in their jackets is the best way – sheer unadulterated goodness. It is little wonder that the Irish got so hooked on them that when a fungus disease took hold of the crop, half the population died of starvation or were forced to emigrate. The fungal problem was so great that scientists returned to the native home of the Murphy, or common spud, in South American to seek some source of immunity to this disease. They found the genes still safe in the diversity of some six thousand or so varieties that had been developed by the people of the Andes long before the Spanish conquered what was left of the Inca civilisation.

As leprosy does not occur in those countries where the potato is a staple in the diet, the introduction of potatoes into Britain by Walter Raleigh is thought to be responsible for the disappearance here of this dreaded disease. Potatoes are not fattening, as many people are led to believe: any fattening is due to the oil or fat in which they are saturated before frying, or the butter or cream added when presented at table. (The British Potato Council recently revealed that the British prefer potato mash to chips!) Statistics show that regular homemade mash is infinitely healthier in calorific, fat and saturates values than processed or bought versions. Potato is highly absorbent and able to soak up up to one-third of its weight in fat – so be warned! Recent research using animals has found that raw potato starch lowers cholesterol and improves mineral retention, and potato extract even looks promising as an anticarcinogenic against malignant mammary cells.

Potato juice can be useful, taken in moderation, for peptic ulcers, alleviating pain and acidity. Mashed pulp is considered a serviceable remedy for external application to painful joints and skin rashes. Sliced raw potato applied to a burn brings relief, as does grated raw potato bound to the area with gauze. Potato water is good for cleaning silver, and its juice added to fuller's earth makes an excellent face mask to remove urban dirt and grease. In India, potato skins are used to treat swollen gums and burns.

SOYA BEAN
Glycine max

ASIA

Soya is one of the few foodstuffs that contain all twenty-two amino acids, the body's building-blocks, necessary to human life;

it also contains 40 per cent protein, 20 per cent fat, 2 per cent lecithin, and vitamins A, B and E, and so meets the criterion for a complete food. The soya bean was referred to in Chinese materia medica over 4,500 years ago. A native to South-West Asia and a plant of generally warm temperate regions, soya has been grown in China, according to the records, for five thousand years. It was not used in the western hemisphere until the late nineteenth century, and first imported into England in 1908. Today the USA grows 60 per cent of the world's 110-million-tonne harvest of this crucially important oil seed crop. The rest is grown in China, Japan and Brazil. Sometimes called 'boneless meat', before cooking dried soya beans contain huge amounts of potassium, phosphorus and iron, large amounts of calcium and magnesium, and relatively high amounts of zinc, manganese and copper and, in particular, selenium and iodine. Both soya beans and their oil are of momentous importance to all the vegetarians on the planet. The beans provide flour, soya milk and cheese, tofu, tempeh, miso and soy sauce. Although they contain more than four times as many calories as beef their sugars are hardly taken into our bodies, so soya or tofu products are ideal foods for diabetics. Recent research on animals suggests that a soya diet may also play a useful role in reducing neuropathic pain.

The Chinese condiment soy sauce, prepared from fermented beans, dates back to pre-Christian times. In research published in 1995, it was referred to as a 'functional seasoning containing alkaloidal components with the potent preventive effect on thrombus formation' – in other words, it showed the ability to stop blood platelets from aggregating and can help to prevent heart disease. Animal research undertaken in 2001 confirms that the isoflavones in soya may help to prevent atherosclerosis.

Soy sauce and miso are produced from the fermented beans, tofu and tempeh from bean curd, and miso soup is a great way to start the day. Soya milk is a good and, in the case of allergies, may be a life-saving substitute for cow's milk. It can be used in a whole range of dairy-like and bakery products, and in its extruded form it has the appearance and texture of fish and meat, while soya bean sprouts are great eaten raw in their natural state. Chinese healers have used mouldy soya bean curds to treat skin infections since early dynastic times. Could it have been the mould *Penicillium* doing the trick thousands of years before Alexander Fleming made his discovery, or did the curds contain something else, perhaps an anti-allergen? Anyone allergic to soya should not use soya-containing products such as cosmetic creams.

PEANUT
Arachis hypogaea
NEW WORLD

Peanuts originated in Brazil. Today, they are an important world crop, especially in Africa. The plant got its popular name from its pea-shaped flower. It is, however, not a nut but a sort of bean. When the plant finishes flowering and the seeds are set, the pod then automatically bends its stem and burrows under ground to develop. Peanuts in their raw state are highly nutritious, consisting of about 45 per cent oil and 30 per cent protein with valuable amounts of iron and vitamins B and E. Peanut mono-unsaturated oil has a high level of polyunsaturated fatty acids. Cold-pressed oils are worth their extra cost, since commercial peanut oil is almost always refined to a high degree using heat treatments, and any vitamin and mineral content is therefore reduced. It should be noted that allergy to peanuts, which has increased steadily in the West over the past twenty years, can cause anaphylaxis and death. Peanut protein is secreted into the milk of lactating women when they have eaten peanuts, and this may result in the sensitisation of at-risk infants.

Used externally, peanut oil is said to help to alleviate arthritis and rheumatism. The oil's high vitamin E content is useful in its antioxidant action against carcinogens, as the vitamin has the ability to neutralise those potentially dangerous free radicals. Vitamin E has also been shown to protect against cardiovascular disease. Peanut oil contains 13–43 per cent linoleic acid, the parent of GLA (gamma linolenic acid), which helps regulate bodily functions, including the control of cell-to-cell communication and the transmission of signals between nerve cells. It is known that those who suffer from multiple sclerosis lack linoleic acid, and the deficiency is thought to be an important factor in the degenerative nature of the disease. In the 1940s a French scientist isolated the compound oligormeric procyanidin (OPC) from the red skin of the peanut and used it to treat oedema in his wife. Known as Resivit, it became the first vasculo-protective medicine to be sold in France.

3

How Did the World's Medicine Get the Way It Is?

People are not unique in doing their best to cure themselves – animals when ill certainly do the same – a fact that soon becomes obvious wherever there are pets within the family unit. The Bellamy household has, or rather had, seven cats. One was ours, an indoor cat of high breeding and well inoculated against the problems of disease. The others we had inherited with the rambling garden, and they all lived outside. The continual struggle of five of them centred on attaining the status of indoor cat, so they were petted and wormed each in due season.

The seventh, called Panda, was a wild individualist, unapproachable by all except one of my children and then only at arm's length. It was great to watch arthritic, ageing Panda, always first to, and king of, the warmest sun-soaked spot. When suffering from a flu-like malaise he would only take cold water and part of his routine was to chew grass and vomit. Only in his last days did he come into the house, where he was consoled not only by the Bellamy clan but by all the cats too, until he passed away purring – a toothless veteran of self-survival in a society overflowing with hygienic cat-lit, worm powders and all the other paraphernalia of twentieth-century peticare.

People, whether they like cats or not, are also social animals. Since their eruption here on earth, the family and gradually the larger social groups have been their units of survival and an important adjunct to their immune system. When a member of the family or a friend bled, they would do their best to stop the bleeding; when burned, they would cool the pain; when cold, the patient would be kept warm, and when hot with fever, kept cool. Illness would often climax with vomiting or diarrhoea; some would recover. Loved ones or important members of the family or clan would have been given the best food available, flavoured with herbs or spices to take away the taste of nausea and the smell of the sickroom. So as new foods were tried and tested, the knowledge of which made you throw up or explosively defecate would be stored away for future use, a quick kill or cure.

Those mums, wives, widows, aunts and their male kin who absorbed more of the local plant lore than others would have been in great demand in the clan or tribe. Success would have engendered both praise and jealousy; protectionism of knowledge, and failure, would have brought claims of witchcraft. The most sought-after of these self-taught physicians may well have been individuals who had themselves recovered from symptoms from which all others had died. He or she may have been desperately ill, even comatose for some time, all hope gone, and then suddenly miraculously recovered. Seeking an explanation themselves, they may have quoted dream experiences from that comatose state and so the whole concept of the witch doctor, the healing shaman, could have arisen.

Recovery from epileptic attacks could have played a similar role. The linking of healing with some form of mystic, religious belief must have been there from the start. There must have been a belief that there was something, someone, out there that could help, and a soul within that was worthy of being helped even after death, for ritualistic burials predate modern humanity.

It could well be that the shaman, the healer, was the first focal point for the bonding of families into clans, and that that same shaman presented medicine with its first dichotomy – between the family herbalist who used the plants to hand, upon which all had come to rely, and the shaman with his or her 'sacred' plants with curative properties, some of which could open psychotic windows on to the supernatural.

Half a millennium before the birth of Christ, over a period of no more than 120 years, five great thinkers were flourishing in different parts of the world. The remarkable thing is that they all came to startlingly similar conclusions regarding people and the living world upon which we all depend and of which we are a part. These thinkers were Zarathustra, Deutero-Isaiah, Siddhartha Gautama the Buddha, Confucius and Pythagoras. History would argue that they never met and in all probability had no knowledge of each other's teachings.

However, Old World trade routes were busy at that time and materia medica – the substances used for healing and their multiform applications – was certainly on the move, so they may well have had knowledge of each other's teachings. The fantastic thing was that, though expressing it in different ways, each came to 'The attainment by an individual human being of a direct personal relation with the ultimate reality in and behind the universe in which man finds himself.' (Toynbee, *Mankind and Mother Earth*). It was from this realisation that evolved the great spiritual philosophies of the world, Brahminism, Buddhism, Christianity, Islam, Judaism, Taoism, Zoroastrianism and Pythagoreanism in all their diverse forms. I quote from Freeman Dyson, Professor of Physics at the University of Princeton, a recent winner of the Templeton Prize for Progress in Religion:

> Science and religion are but two windows that people look through, trying to understand the big universe outside, trying to understand why we are here. The two windows give different views, but they look out at the same universe. Both views are one-sided, neither is complete. Both leave out essential features of the real world. And both are worthy of respect. Science and religion should work together to abolish the gross inequalities that prevail in the modern world. That is my vision, and it is the same vision that inspired Francis Bacon four hundred years ago, when he prayed that through science God would 'endow the human family with new mercies'.

In eastern Asia and elsewhere in the Orient, shamanism and animism predate the more familiar mainstream religious philosophies of Buddhism and Confucianism. Yet despite the fact that ecstatics, shamans and diviners were banished when Confucianism was established as the state religion in China two thousand years ago and during the cultural revolution, shamanic vestiges remain in the Taoist tradition, which is still served by monasteries and temples throughout the country.

An interesting story to which the Borneo Dayaks refer in their legends is of a somewhat shamanic journey to the sky. The god Tupa-Jing noticed that the Dayaks were on the verge of destroying themselves because they had no cures for sickness, and were cremating ill people out of necessity. He therefore saved a woman from the funeral pyre as she ascended in clouds of smoke, took her to heaven, and instructed her in the skills of medicine. With these, she was able to return to earth and pass on the precious knowledge she had obtained. From the New World comes the account of the Chumash medicine woman Chequeesh, who told anthropologist Will Noffke in 1985 that she had learned of her native heritage by utilising the 'dream herb', mugwort (*Artemisia vulgaris*). Then again, for the Jivaro of Ecuador the familiar world is a lie or an illusion and there is only one reality, that of the supernatural – a reality on to which a window may be opened by using certain plants which have come to be known as hallucinogenic and which, at least in the modern world, have given a whole new and sinister meaning to the word 'drug'.

The arguments about the rights and wrongs of ritualistic medicine and of the use and abuse of psychoactive drugs will continue as long as there are people and plants left on this earth. However that may be, over the millennia and down the centuries the local herbal practitioner must have continued to do a good job, making use of everything that was to hand and so doing Trojan work for human society. Herbal medicine was here to stay.

There are, of course, no written accounts of the origins of the herbalist or the shaman, but there is some archaeological evidence. This comes to us in the form of burials in which the internee had been laid to rest prepared for the afterlife, with food and medicine – grave goods that link both the practice and the profession of herbalism with the mystery of eternity.

The most ancient evidence unearthed to date that links the concept of an afterlife with herbal healing comes from the country we now call Iraq and from a district with the haunting name of Shanidar. There some sixty thousand years ago a man of Neanderthal lineage was put to rest in a shallow grave which already contained the remains of two adult females and a baby. The soil, which had so long enclosed his bones, bore the tell-tale pollen grains of plants that still grow in abundance in the woods and fields around the grave site, and the grains of eight of the plants were in such great abundance that they must have been placed in the grave with the bodies. It may well be that the grave flowers were no more than decoration and had no medical significance, but as some were spring- and some were summer-flowering they must have been stored ready for use. Add to that the fact that seven of the plants are used to this day in the herbal medicine of the locality, and all appeared in the *British Pharmacopoeia* of the mid-twentieth century, a vast tome listing all the known plants used across the ten thousand years that saw the births of all the civilisations. These civilisations had been served well enough by organic food and herbal medicine in all their forms to allow the human population to cross the 1.5 billion mark.

A SHORT HISTORY OF HERBAL MEDICINE*

12,000–5000 BC

In the warmer parts of the world away from the main effects of the ice age, human society and the medicine upon which it came to depend developed more rapidly than in more temperate climes. At first, the knowledge and practice of herbal healing must have evolved through trial and error, and there must have been some painful and catastrophic results. No doubt the hunting people watched animals very closely and learned from them. For example, just as our pet cats and dogs will eat certain plants to make them sick, so do wild animals. If bitten by a snake, chamois deer are known to graze on distasteful spurges, which give them violent diarrhoea; wolves appear to dig up and eat the root of bistort for the same reason. Muskrats will coat wounds with resin that they gather from pine trees. Today, we have some evidence that hinds eat certain species of lily to bring themselves on heat, while some apes and monkeys browse on specific types of leaves and fruits which 'regulate' conception.

Such knowledge, once gleaned, would have been passed down the family line of 'herb women', grandmother to granddaughter. Then probably as chauvinism came to rule some roosts, the simple knowledge became entangled in the rites and wrongs of shamanistic religion, with all its professional jealousies.

* Adapted from my book *Blooming Bellamy*, published by BBC Enterprises.

From 2000 BC to the classical period

In the second millennium BC medical papyri were being written in Egypt recording the use of more than 260 plants, and in Assyria similar information concerning 250 medicines was put on record on tablets of clay.

Sometime in the second century BC the *Atharva-Veda*, containing much herbal law and folk medicine, was handed to Brahma, the supreme Hindu god, in India. In Israel, the Talmud and the Old Testament were written, both containing many references to health practice and some to herbal medicine. The Koran, written by the followers of Islam during the Prophet Mohammed's lifetime (c.570–632), contains similar good news, giving us an insight into the wonder of the great civilisations that developed in North Africa and along the shores of the Mediterranean. Also in the first century AD, Shen Nong, the mythical Divine Peasant of China, began to compile his *Great Herbal*.

Greek legend has it that the doctor Asklepios was so good at healing the sick that the chief god, Zeus, became jealous and killed him with a thunderbolt. Later, temple hospitals called *asklepieia* were built in healthful places in the countryside near springs and streams. People came to these temples to worship the god of healing – which Asklepios had become, at the recommendation of Apollo – and to seek cures. Priests looked after the patients, bathing them and putting them on a diet. When the priests thought the time was right, they took the individual to a special room in the temple, the *abaton*, where he was given drugs such as poppy seeds or hemlock. At first, the patients left gifts in the temple for Asklepios, but later many of the priests began to demand money. As late as 293 BC the Romans began to worship Asklepios, building a temple to him on an island in the middle of the River Tiber.

About this time similar things were happening in Sri Lanka, where we find the first records of hospitals and convalescent homes built by Buddhist monks between 397 and 307 BC. A little later Asoka, King of India, helped to develop systems of law, order and medicine throughout the country (264–223 BC). The medicine practised in the subcontinent in the first seven hundred years AD was summarised in the *Charaka Samhita* and *Susruta Samhita*, two great works that became the main foundations of Ayurvedic medicine, which still serves many people well to this day.

The Greek physician Hippocrates is said to have been born around 400 BC on Kos, now better known as a Greek holiday island. Because so little is known about him, some scholars say he probably never existed, but a school of medicine that bore his name definitely did. It gave the world much herbal knowledge, as well as the Hippocratic oath of ethical conduct. Its members were the fathers of therapeutic medicine. Theophrastus, today recognised as the 'Father of Botany', was a Greek philosopher born on the island of Lesbos around 372 BC and dying in Athens some eighty-five years later. Dioscorides, who lived during the first century AD, was born in Cilicia. He penned a gigantic tome called *De Materia Medica* that listed more than five hundred plants and became the main textbook of Western herbal medicine for the next thousand years. He also sowed the seeds of the 'Doctrine of Signatures', the theory suggesting that plants which looked like parts of the human body would help cure afflictions of those parts. Then there was Galen, who was born in Pergamum in Greece around 130 AD and died in Italy seventy years later. He was regarded as the 'Father of Pharmacy', and his main work, *De Simplicibus*, was a standard medical text in the Arab and Western world until the Renaissance. Some of his prescriptions are still in use today.

The Middle Ages

During the Tang dynasty the Chinese government commissioned one Su Ying to write the official *Tang Materia Medica*. Completed around 659 AD, its fifty-four volumes overflowed with descriptions of the many plants used in Chinese medicine. Charlemagne, King of the Franks and Emperor of the West, was born around 742 AD at Neustria in northern France and died at Aachen at the age of sixty-two. He or his son issued a number of Acts or laws, one of which listed that plants should be grown on the royal estates. The most famous of Islam's physicians is certainly Rhazes, born in Ravy around 865 AD. He died sixty years later, having completed a prodigious amount of work still of great use today, with many of the plant species he recommended still used in the formulation of modern medicines.

Around 900 AD the manual of a Saxon doctor was written down in his own language. Called *The Leech Book of Bald*, it is the earliest European herbal written in the vernacular. During the next century lived Avicenna, one of the most famous men of the Arab world, who came to be known as the 'Prince of Physicians'. Born in 980 AD, he died in Hamadan in Persia in 1037 having written his amazing *Canon of Medicine*, still in use today. An Arab traveller of the same century expressed amazement at the availability of oriental spices in Rhineland markets, proving that the trade routes were already open to herbal medicine, as well as to diseases like the Black Death which followed on.

St Hildegard, born in Germany in 1098, led a life of saintly service creating and developing a physic garden at the Convent of Rupertsberg near Bingen, where she died in 1179.

The legend of the Physicians of Myddfai has it that a farm boy successfully courted and married a lady who appeared one day, complete with dowry, out of a lake in South Wales. Having returned to the lake, she later reappeared and gave her three sons a packet of herbal prescriptions, which were put to good use for the next thousand years. Fortunately for generations of rural people and for the princes of South Wales, the prescriptions used by the Physicians of Myddfai were written down for posterity sometime in the thirteenth century.

Meanwhile, some three hundred miles to the north, near Soutra on the Lammamuir hills south of Edinburgh on route to England, a large hospital was at work serving the local monastic community and the many travellers who used the road. Recent excavation has unearthed large quantities of hospital waste that, in the dedicated hands of Dr Brian Moffat and his co-workers, is revealing detailed and fascinating information about medieval medicine. Despite the fact that the Soutra hospital, one of more than a thousand then operating in Britain, was situated some 335 metres above sea level, the monks grew three very important drug plants, probably in walled gardens: flax, hemp and the opium poppy. They also made use of tormentil, a native plant that grew and still grows in abundance thereabouts.

Around 1250 AD, *De Proprietatibus Rerum* by Bartholomaeus Anglicus was written. This was a truly amazing nineteen volumes of natural history, the seventeenth of which constituted the only original herbal written in England during the Middle Ages. A little later the London Guilds of Pepperers and Spicers joined forces to become the

Fraternity of St Anthony, an unholy alliance that included the apothecaries. By the mid-1400s they had taken on the collective name of Grocers, and together profited from the spice wars and the bloody European expansion.

1500–1900 The age of 'heroic medicine' and herbals

With the advent of printing about 1454, the scarce manuscripts of the past, which contained handwritten details of herbs and herbal medicines, were soon published. The knowledge they contained, both accurate and inaccurate, was made available to anyone who cared to learn to read and could afford the luxury of books.

Philippus Aureolus Theophrastus Bombastus von Hohenheim, known as Paracelsus, was the son of a Swiss physician and was born in 1493 near Einsiedel. In his youth he witnessed the problems caused by the effects of mercury and other poisons on the miners and their families who worked in and around the local metal and mineral mines. At medical school he became a rebel, counselling the wise use of all medicines and pointing out the need for correct dosage in each case. If only more people had taken notice of his pleas, many would have been saved extreme suffering, for the 'kill or cure', or 'heroic' medicine, became mainstream at that time, and medical practitioners came to rely on too frequent use of many poisons such as mercury and antimony.

But while many mainstream doctors and quacks came to rely on too frequent blood-letting, a practice taught in the medical schools of the day, as well as on ultra-violent emetics and purges and small but regular doses of deadly poisons that did their patients more harm than good, others continued to work wonders with plants. Among these were many of the womenfolk, from the humblest cottage to the grandest residence. Gervase Markham's *The English Housewife*, first published in 1615, set down much homespun wisdom. It ran to many editions and was a bestseller throughout the century. Markham acknowledged the fact that much of the contents of the book was taken from a manuscript which had belonged to Lady Frances, Countess Dowager of Exeter.

The first English-language herbal was by Richard Banckes. Published in 1525, it was in essence a copy of manuscripts of the fourteenth century, a link with the Physicians of Myddfai. It includes a poem on the virtues of seventy-seven herbs, and the famous discourse on rosemary sent by the French Countess of Hainault to her daughter, Philippa (c. 1314–69), Edward III's queen. Back in those days good news about herbal medicine travelled fast, and none faster than *Joyfull Newes Out of the Newe Founde Worlde* by Nicolas Monardes, a Spanish doctor, published in 1569. This was the first American herbal, providing information on the herbs then flowing into Europe from the Americas, and appeared in English, Latin, Italian, Flemish and French. The year 1590 saw the publication of a *Compendium of Materia Medica* by the Chinese physician Li Shi Zhen. Its fifty-two volumes describing nearly two thousand drugs, mainly of plant origin, were revised in 1765 by one Zhao Xue Min, who added a further nine hundred.

At that time herbals were coming off the presses thick and fast, and few were thicker than that of John Gerard. Called 'the greate herball', its 1,630 huge pages containing more than half a million words came complete with illustrations and was first published in 1597. Despite its many faults, mistakes and plagiarisms, this *Herball, or Generall Historie of Plants* became the standard work for English students. John Parkinson was another herbalist of the grand tradition, for he ran a lucrative and fashionable practice while at the same time keeping a physic garden to supply his clients' herbal needs. On the title-page of his herbal *Paradisus Terrestris* (published in 1629) he linked the two in a pun on his name – *Paradisi in Sole* (meaning 'Park in Sun').

In those days, the hierarchy of healing ran something like this. At the top were the physicians, whose formal training at the universities of Oxford and Cambridge could last fourteen years. There they presided, steeped in the classical works and the complexities of materia medica. Then came the surgeons, who in the absence of anaesthetics were performing their many operations at lightning speed. Then came the barber surgeons who did the blood-letting and tooth extraction, and finally the apothecaries, who kept up the supply of vegetables, minerals and even animals that went into the pills and potions.

Nicholas Culpeper is without doubt the best-known English apothecary of all time. Herbalist, astrologer and doctor, he published in 1651 the first English translation of *The London Dispensatory*. Until that time this pharmacopoeia had been published only in Latin by the self-important College of Physicians, most of whose members did not like their secrets being revealed in a language that the general public could understand. The book is still in print to this day, and many herbal stores still carry his name and his tradition of healing.

SUFFERING PATIENTS, PROFESSIONAL FEUDING, AND PROGRESS AT LAST

During the Industrial Revolution, things went from bad to worse. The countryside could no longer provide unlimited gainful employment for the exploding population, so more and more people were forced to live in the crowded conditions of the new towns. There they had no access to the traditional herbal cures of the countryside and they could not afford the prices charged by the physicians and apothecaries, who were few in number and therefore in great demand. John Wesley (1703–91), a Methodist preacher without equal, became the people's champion. His little pamphlet *Primitive Physic, or A Natural and Easy Method of Curing Most Diseases*, published in 1781, preached good sense and the use of cheap and easily obtained plant remedies, some even from the native peoples of North America.

William Withering (1741–99) graduated in medicine from Edinburgh University steeped in mainstream practice and malpractice. However, he knew that many of the old herbal cures had worked well over the centuries as well as understanding the danger of medicines made from very poisonous plants. To help solve what was an ongoing problem, he carried out pioneer, now classic, research to check the plants and regularise the preparation and dosages of the medicines. His work led to the great corpus of research-based knowledge in which pharmaceutical science has its foundations, work that later formed the basic content of the great tomes known as *The British Pharmacopoeia* and The *Pharmaceutical Codex*. These were continuously updated, and purported to contain the best knowledge and practice at the date of publication.

In Germany, Christian Friedrich Samuel Hahnemann, a brilliant linguist and chemist, graduated in medicine in 1799. Finding that he could bring on the symptoms of a number of fevers by dosing himself with certain herbs or herbal extracts, he developed the idea of homoeopathy, the use of minute amounts of herbal extracts to speed the body into the condition being treated and so into the body's natural cycle of healing.

Just as John Wesley and others had brought back interesting news of herbal medicine as practised by the indigenous people of North America, with the increase in transatlantic travel other good news began to spread fast. Samuel Thompson (1769–1843), the son of a poor farmer from New Hampshire, became a champion of herbal medicine across the world. He too was an advocate of the traditional remedies of the Native North Americans and especially of their 'steam-bath' techniques of aromatherapy. *A Narrative of the Life and Medical Discoveries of Samuel Thompson*, published in 1825, gives a fascinating insight into the practices of these times.

At the start of the nineteenth century, about 20 per cent of the people of England and Wales lived in towns of over five thousand inhabitants. One hundred years later, the figure was nearer 80 per cent. Urbanisation had arrived; but would it turn out to be the only hope for servicing the needs of an exploding population – or the scourge of humanity? Whatever the answer, it had come to stay, and by the end of the twentieth century a lifetime in the city would be the lot of more than 60 per cent of the world's people.

The problems were then, as they remain, to maintain the supply of an adequate healthful diet and of potable water, and the disposal of human waste, which back in the 1800s meant just faeces and urine, for society as a whole was not rich enough to disown rubbish. At the input end of the problem great institutions like Covent Garden and Smithfield markets did their best to supply the populace with food, and ships of many lines scoured the Empire for food and its seabird colonies for fertiliser. At the output end of the line (about eleven metres of it in the case of a grown man), rivers like the Thames became open sewers, dangerous to live near let alone win an election beside. (In the big stinks of the 1850s, blankets soaked in phenol were hung up at the windows of the Palace of Westminster to keep the hot air in and the foetid air out.) The most readily available water supply was thus rendered unfit for any consumption; some of it was so ripe, so charged with organic matter, that one of the few uses to which it could be put was to brew it into beer at Wapping, the alcohol content rendering it safe to drink. There must have been many good men and true within the medical establishment who did their best against the rising tide of urban disease. But the truth of the matter was that there weren't enough medics and there wasn't enough knowledge to go round.

Albert Isaiah Coffin (1790–1866) was born in America, but he decided to cross the Atlantic and was soon popularising the cause of botanic medicine across the length and breadth of Britain. He found a friend and colleague in one John Skelton, a herbalist from Plymouth who had learned the laws of his healing profession from his grandmother, a doctress and midwife in the village of Holberton in Devon, where he was born in 1806. Together they provided much needed help to some of the millions who crowded the industrial cityscapes of those times, battling against epidemics of cholera and worse. Together, and later alone and embittered through jealousy of each other's success, along with others they spawned many local societies such as the Eclectic, Botanic, Medical and Phrenological Institute of Derby.

The medical establishment, perceiving their professional status jeopardised, hated these unqualified upstarts' every move and trained all their guns in their direction. But they were on the losing side: the Coffinites were filling the widening gaps in healthcare with more humane treatments and remedies at more humane prices, and on many occasions these treatments were seen to work. The advice they gave also made great sense: 'Don't purge the newborn with castor oil, let alone calomel [mercury]'; 'Don't lance gums to ease the natural process of teething'; 'Feed them with breast milk, it's nature's way'; 'When constipated, regulate your diet and eat rye bread'; 'Corsets and drugs are no good for rickets. Let the children have fresh air, good food and take plenty of exercise in the open air.' These were the basic tenets of Coffinism, rammed home at every opportunity in lecture, pamphlet and journal, and few people would disagree with any of them today.

Coffin also took up the cry against the use of laudanum, which was at that time being sold for all manner of purposes from all manner of outlets. It found a special use for keeping babies quiet. In Nottingham one member of the town council sold four hundred gallons of laudanum a year; no wonder the pharmacists of the day were called 'druggists'. Opium by any other name would be as addictive, and it was so widely used that Mrs Beeton gave advice for dealing with overdoses in many editions of her famous books on household management.

No wonder, either, that infant mortality rose to 67 per cent in the

1800s in some towns of northern England, where working mothers clubbed together to employ communal wet-nurses to mind their children so that they could return to the loom immediately after giving birth. Women, men and children were working in appalling conditions, their newborn generation of workers crushed into crowded rooms, their dark lives rarely touched by the sun. Children suffered from rickets, and exhausted baby-minders and parents alike turned to the soporific effect of opium to quell the cries of their sick offspring so that they could obtain a good night's sleep or a midday nap. Dr Coffin was one strong voice among many that railed against the inadequacies of the law as regarded opium, and in 1868 the Pharmacy Act was passed, which allowed it to be sold only by qualified pharmacists.

Unfortunately for the cause of herbalism, Albert Isaiah Coffin succumbed to the same problems of human nature: envy and jealousy, which also afflicted his nowadays never-mentioned mentor John Skelton. Quarrelling among the new breeds of botanical medics who burgeoned in the wake of Coffin's immense success opened gaps in the armour of all their arguments: gaps revealing wounds that the establishment blistered and bled to their hearts' content. Within the ranks of the herbalists there were quacks of the worst sort, but botanical medicine should have come through the ordeal in much better shape than it did, for many strong voices within the profession were warning of the problems incurred by calomel and blood-letting and all the other excesses of heroic medicine. Florence Nightingale described as a common sight 'a great-grandmother who was a tower of physical vigour descending into a grandmother perhaps a little less vigorous, but sound as a bell and healthy to the core, into a mother languid and confined to her carriage and house, and lastly into a daughter sickly and confined to her bed'.

About the same time in America Dr Worthington Hooker, commenting on the current state of medicine, declared in a widely publicised prize-winning *Essay on Rational Therapeutics*: 'The deliverance from the suffering that formerly came from fruitless medication is of itself no small gain. The amount of life saved [by that fruitless medication] would be seen to be very small if only we could obtain correct statistics.' In the more forthright words of Oliver Wendell Holmes to the Massachusetts Medical Society in 1860: 'I honestly believe that if the whole *materia medica* [apart from opium and a small number of specific drugs] as now used could be sunk to the bottom of the sea, it would be all the better for mankind – and all the worse for the fishes.'

The medical profession just had to pull its socks up and, among other remedial measures, bring their dose rates down. They began to do just that: by 1870 the *Buffalo Medical and Surgical Journal*, for example, could state: 'Men of high reputation in the profession rely mostly on nature and hygiene.'

NATURE AND HYGIENE

The use of soil in the earth closet, or garden privy, to which fresh earth was added to cover the faeces certainly dealt with the nasty smells. This led to extensive experimentation by the Revd Henry Moule of Fordington, Dorsetshire, and Dr Adinnell Hewson of the Pennsylvania Hospital. Their research highlighted the fact that earth not only did away with the odours produced by gangrene and other diseases, but also brought about miraculous cures of a range of diseases, even of smallpox, a fact published in the *Pacific Medical and Surgical Journal* in November 1869. Why these techniques were not further developed we can only guess; pride and prejudice must have ranked high on the list of possible explanations, and the fact remains that even back in those days it was impossible to patent Mother Earth.

The cholera epidemics of the early 1800s which swept the urbanising world found the medical profession entirely wanting: bleeding and purging simply weakened the patient and hastened the dire symptoms. Here again the botanical medicorps had to come to their aid. For instance, in America the homoeopathic use of camphor by the hourly drop was such a success that it became top of the drops during those worrying times. At first ridiculing the remedy, the medical profession eventually had to admit to a convention of the American Medical Association that camphor had been one of the most valuable remedies used in the treatment of cholera. Meanwhile in England, Coffin published daily accounts of his successes and others' failures in his *Bulletin of Health*.

It was, however, the brilliant detective work of Dr John Snow that in 1854 traced the source of what, thanks to him, became London's last cholera epidemic. Though others scoffed at the idea of such a virulent disease being carried by water, when Snow removed the handle from what his research had shown to be the offending pump in Broadwick Street in Soho, the scourge of cholera was conquered. From that momentous day on, it was up to the civil engineers and scientists to direct their awesome powers to the problem, and they solved it by using simple sand filters backed up by steam pumps – layers of clean sand that effectively filtered out the microbes, producing pure water.

It was to be the era of wrought-iron and marble palaces of cleanliness. The first modern national health systems were thus gradually put in place, and the disease and death rates began to fall away. The decline in tuberculosis in the second half of the century was entirely due to the improvements in hygiene, which also accounted for about half the decline in the death rate over that period. It cannot be denied that the Victorian era, for all its faults, was responsible for that huge breakthrough, the flush lavatory, with its substructure of cathedral-like sewers, their branches reaching out to every source of potential corruption. Vast numbers of labourers built vast works that collected and discharged the sewage into rivers and estuaries below the towns' water intakes. These stupendous feats of civil and civilising engineering, though out of sight and so out of mind, deserve world heritage status just as much as the pyramids of Egypt or the cities on the ancient spice routes. As does the handle of the pump in Broadwick Street, London W1.

Throughout the later nineteenth century, besides sanitation and public hygiene, one other factor appeared to be making major inroads into the death toll due to disease: it was called 'immunisation'. A hundred years previously heroes like Jan Ingenhousz and Thomas Dimsdale had risked more than their reputations when summoned to inoculate some of Europe's most powerful royal dynasties against smallpox, using dried pus from the pustules of patients infected by the disease. And in 1798, thirty years later, the first vaccine was produced by Edward Jenner, the British physician who found that the virus of cowpox (*Vaccinia*) when inoculated into humans could provide lasting protection against one of our most ancient and disfiguring diseases. And thanks to the pioneer work of Louis Pasteur, which culminated in the acceptance of the germ theory of disease, the sciences of bacteriology, virology and immunology came into being.

The arguments both for and against immunisation have waxed and waned for over two hundred years, as have the arguments for and against both orthodox medicine and traditional herbal medicine. Vested interests, notwithstanding Hippocratic oaths and age-old traditions, will justify or vilify the means long before any end is in sight.

It was in 1877 that Jesse Boot, having given up the presidency of the Eclectic, Botanic, Medical and Phrenological Institute of Derby, opened his first chemist's shop in Nottingham. Later he began to manufacture drugs on a large scale, then set up his own empire of Boots Cash Chemists. In his own words, penned later: 'I thought the public would welcome new chemists' shops in which a greater and a better variety of pharmaceutical articles could be bought at cheaper prices.' Whether he was influenced in this by the arguments of splinter groups within the herbal movement, by the increasing cost of importing the Eclectic herbal concentrates from America, or by the pressures exerted by the new science of chemotherapeutics, is not clear. Whatever his motivation, Sir Jesse brought modern pharmaceutics to the high street and, sadly, he and his wife declined their invitation to the opening of the British Herbal Association School in September 1911.

THE AGE OF CHEMOTHERAPEUTICS

Chemotherapeutics, the use of specific chemicals directed at a specific pathogen or cancer, is said to have begun when Mithradates VI, King of Pontus (120–63 BC) on the Black Sea, out of fear of being poisoned, experimented with both animal and vegetable poisons and tried to immunise himself by taking increasing (but sublethal) dosages of poisons he had tested on his slaves. The whole affair backfired when, defeated repeatedly by Rome and under siege by his own mutinous troops led by his son, he tried to commit suicide by poisoning – and failed miserably, so that he had to order one of his mercenaries to kill him. Out of this came the whole sad argument for and against using animals to test the efficacy and safety of drugs, new and old – an argument that will probably go on as long as there are people who have never watched a loved one or a beloved pet suffer from a terminal illness.

The greatest revolution in world medicine for over two thousand years began with the work of Paul Erlich (1854–1915): it was called 'chemotherapeutics'. Involving himself early in his career in studies in immunity, Erlich developed the theory that immunity depended on specifically adapted side-chains on protein molecules. He also showed that immunity to toxic substances in mice could be increased many thousandfold by a slowly increasing exposure to them. He eventually developed an organic compound of arsenic for combating the bacteria present in syphilis and yaws: 'Salvarsan' (a.k.a. '606') was ready in 1910 and became available for general use after the first large-scale medical tests to prove the suitability for use in humans of what was suspected to be a potentially toxic substance.

Until then, testing had been a long-term trial-and-error process that had eventually come up with adequate but not excessive dosages which every student of pharmacy had to learn by rote. It was in part his or her job and liability to check the dosage on those hurriedly scribbled prescriptions, as a double check against errors that might prove fatal. With never-before-heard-of substances appearing on the market, the thousands of years of trial-and-error testing had to be circumscribed by laboratory tests involving the use – unethical, however well regulated, in the eyes of some – of millions of animals.

The human organism, far from perfect in both the physical and the moral sense, was open to all sorts of infections both acute and chronic, and there was then still none more worrying than syphilis. Mercury worked for some, but caused havoc for others. So it was not surprising when the new wonder drug, Salvarsan, soon showed up side-effects too: jaundice, kidney disease, optic atrophy, anaphylactic shock and arsenical dermatitis, which could skin the bloated patient alive. The pleas of the National Association of Medical Herbalists that, using herbal remedies, they had successfully cured thousands of cases of syphilis in all its stages went unheeded, as legislation was passed that made it illegal for any but qualified medical practitioners to treat the disease.

Meanwhile pneumonia, puerperal fever and meningitis were raging through the desperate clientele of those on both sides of the argument. The only difference was that if patients died under the care of a regular physician, few questions would be asked except perhaps by the physician, whereas if patients died while under the care of a medical herbalist, questions might well be asked at a very expensive Crown inquest. It's therefore surprising to learn that at the outbreak of war in 1914 the Board of Agriculture and Fisheries issued a pamphlet extolling *The Cultivation of Medical Plants in England*. The public response was enormous, and the pamphlet certainly helped fill the gap in the new materia medica that had been in the main imported from the Continent.

One particularly important product of this herbal home front was onions, to be used as an antiseptic for suppurating wounds. In 1916 the government urgently asked for tons of them, offering the munificent price of 1 shilling a pound, so highly were they prized by the front-line surgeons. They used these odoriferous bulbs to great effect along with the adsorptive and healing power of sphagnum moss, collected from wherever it grew in abundance from Scotland to British Columbia. In the latter region it had long been employed as diapers for Native American babies, who rarely suffered from nappy rash. Another herb that found favour on the front, where gas attacks had occurred, was lily-of-the-valley (*Convallaria majalis*). It was used as a cardiac tonic, for it not only had that smell of garden corners 'that will be forever England' but also produced a digitalis-like effect.

Thanks to these stories of success, the public interest in herbal remedies outlasted the war effort. The result was the setting-up in 1927 of the Society of Herbalists at its headquarters, Culpeper House, Runton Street, London W1. In those days herbalists' shops like that of Potter and Clarke in London's Farringdon Road, presided over by a Miss Oakley, attracted a wide cross-section of customers, as Barbara Griggs so fragrantly records in the classic *Green Pharmacy* (1985).

Office girls anxious to lose weight came in to have made for them a mixture containing bladderwrack (*Fucus vesiculosus*) – that brown rubbery seaweed with the round pod-shaped bubbles which children love to pop – believed to counter obesity by stimulating the thyroid gland. Tired businessmen dropped in for a tonic made out of kola (Cola spp.) – as stimulating as caffeine – and damiana (*Turnera diffusa* var. *aphrodisiaca*) which, as its official name suggests, is believed in Mexico 'to be especially good for tired businessmen'.

However, throughout this time both the herbalists and the regular practitioners had more to worry about than tired businessmen and inquests on the deaths of patients. All, and especially the latter, were open to infection from their own patients. A prick or scratch could bring the terror of systemic infection and even of gas gangrene raging through their own bodies. And so they would perhaps turn to onions, backed up by a handful of blowfly maggots, which had been used with success in the trenches to clean up wounds.

As I write, I am aware of a scar on my left arm where for three agonising weeks during 1939 drainage tubes protruded from a persistent abscess. Then Dad came home from the shop with 'May & Baker 69', one of the new sulphonamide-containing wonder drugs. Twenty-four hours later – no more tubes, no more lancets, no more hot fomentations – my arm was on the mend. At Queen Charlotte's Hospital in London where I was born in 1933 the first sulphonamide, Prontosil Red (researched and developed by Paul Ehrlich), had reduced the death rate from puerperal fever from 20 to 5 per cent. My mother, who had suffered from anaemia during her confinement, had been fed on raw liver, a cure recently discovered along with the role of pancreatic insulin in diabetes. The year 1928 had seen Fleming's miraculous discovery of penicillin and my brother, three years my senior, had been taken to meet one of my father's night-school friends, Lewis Holt, who was working in Fleming's laboratory at St Mary's Hospital in Paddington. He was in fact used as a guinea-pig in Uncle Lewis's research testing a vaccine for catarrh.

The establishment was faced with a problem: either they had to accept that long-term use and re-use gave old plant drugs scientific and legal acceptability, or they had to call for them to be tested with the rigour with which the new synthetic drugs were being tested, and eventually, perhaps, to be labelled with all their contents. They chose the latter course of action. Their excuse was, in part, that if it was expensive to test a single new patentable synthetic chemical, who would bear the cost of testing a herb, with all its complex biochemicals? To test a whole-plant drug, even if it had been used in antiquity, would cost millions; indeed, if one had to list on the packet all the chemicals that give garlic or broccoli their distinctive taste, many of the flavourful components would be regarded, and rightly so, as poisons, for in high concentrations some of them *are* very poisonous.

These were heady times for medicine, and especially for the pharmaceutical industry. For the 'magic bullets' of chemotherapeutic allopathy – orthodox medical practice – appeared to hold the key to universal health and to multinational wealth. Botanic medicine and herbalists began to take on a more folksy and outdated appearance. Almost the only exception was Germany, where despite a very lucrative drug industry Adolf Hitler aided the passing of a law that gave naturopaths and herbalists almost equal status with doctors and surgeons; in France, too, the *herboristes* (herbalists) found increasing state support.

Back in beleaguered Britain things herbal went from bad to worse. The 1941 Pharmacy and Medicines Act removed the right of the National Association of Medical Herbalists to do what they were set up to do: they could no longer legally supply their patients with herbal medicines. They took their complaints and put their pleas for fair play to the highest authority in the land, but all to no avail. More pressing matters overtook the government, for the Second World War demanded penicillin on a massive scale and, thanks to the work of Howard Florey, Ernst Chain and their colleagues, the pharmaceutical industry came up with the goods. They grew *Penicillium chrysogenum* successfully in deep culture, and so when the Allied armies marched in to save Europe, some of them passing by what remained of the ancient medical school at Salerno, at least they were more or less immune from the effects of venereal disease. In this war against an age-old enemy there were deaths and debilitating side-effects, but moral codes could be redrafted, and the age of antibiotics opened the door to streptomycin (isolated from soil), which would be a fierce combatant in the fight. With new biosynthetic and semi-synthetic chemicals now coming on stream, bespoke antibiotics were upon us.

New-age pharmacists and old-age herbalists alike forgot that these were in the main natural products that had been employed in classical times, as recorded in the Ebers papyrus of c. 1500 BC. Of all the twentieth-century developments, antibiotics more than any others should have forged links between herbalism and modern medicine, not new rifts and divisions. Similarly with the new immunisation technique, for it can be looked on as no more than an extension of the natural process of passive immunisation whereby, for example, primate and rodent foetuses (via the placenta) and hoofed animals (via the colostrum) gain immunity from their mothers, at least for the first vital months of their lives. If the connection had been made and the knowledge put to creative use, perhaps Aneurin Bevan, visionary statesman that he was, when drafting plans for the National Health Service would have included the herbalists within its remit. The fact that he didn't is hard to understand, because in the post-war years there was good news on the herbal medicine front. Many of the pharmaceutical companies appeared to be turning away from the 'magic bullet' approach of chemotherapy towards reinvestigating at least some of those 'impure' whole plants.

As I mentioned earlier, my dad was a pharmacist, manager of the local branch of Boots Cash Chemists, back in the days before antibiotics and modern drugs really hit the scene. His shop had dozens of drawers made of mahogany, each with an ivory handle (the world didn't worry about such things in those days). Each drawer contained parts of plants – roots, leaves, buds, stems, flowers, fruits and seeds: the materia medica that formed the basis of most of the medicines, powders, pills, extracts, tinctures, tisanes, electuaries (medicines mixed with syrup) and suppositories that he dispensed across the counter. Then, my dad was an important part of a real national health system, translating prescriptions hastily scribbled by overworked doctors into pills and potions. He would recommend proprietary brands, always emphasising that the instructions on the packet must be followed to the T while counselling that, yes, little Jenny was bad enough to warrant the expense of going to the doctor's.

It was all very well to argue that with the whole herb you got the whole tonic package, including the active living principle of cytoplasm, sap and roughage, while the chemically produced drugs were a much simpler thing, in many cases a single type of molecule, and so more readily caused allergies in the patient and greater resistance in the pathogen. Shades of super bugs to come. Sadly, the establishment took little notice.

A GREEN RENAISSANCE

It was therefore remarkable that in the 1920s, in the middle of the chemotherapeutic revolution, one of the biggest drug houses in

America, Eli Lilley, began marketing a herbal remedy that was both a useful decongestant for asthma and a stimulant of the central nervous system. This was ephedrine, the active constituent of the joint pine (*Ephedra*), the pollen of which had lain so long in that grave in Shanidar (see p 57). In 1942 Harold Randall Griffith and G. Enid Johnson were opening up new vistas in heart surgery with the use of curare as a muscle relaxant – a major and exciting breakthrough. But curare, extracted from the vines and lianas found growing in tropical rainforests, had been used for millennia by Amerindian tribes as a fish and an arrow poison. At the same time, at the height of the Second World War just as the Philippines were falling to the Japanese, Colonel Arthur F. Fisher, wracked with malaria, smuggled seeds of cultivated cinchona out of Java to America, whence the trees' ancestors had come.

Malaria was one of the main enemies in that particular theatre of war, and at the time Java produced the world's best cinchona bark, the only source then of the only prophylactic for the disease. With no time to set up plantations in the West, a true-life adventure began high in the Andes. Led by American botantist Dr William C. Steer, a motley band of adventurers set out to source adequate supplies of quinine, contained in the bark. At altitudes where equatorial hypothermia is a silent night-time killer, these unsung heroes found the precious cinchona trees growing on precipitous cliffs. Locating, harvesting and transporting the wet bark was a nightmare that opened up the terrain to massive erosion and the workers to a plethora of diseases. They also found, like Nicholas Culpeper and William Withering before them, that biological variation was a problem. Not only did the different species of cinchona tree give different yields but, also, different stands of the same species showed immense variation in the amount of quinine, cinchonine, cinchonidine and quinidine they contained. The latter was then in great demand for use in treating certain types of heart disease, and the other three were used in the manufacture of totaquine, a seminatural product that is still a successful antimalarial even when many of the more modern synthetic prophylactics are losing their clout.

These fieldworkers found that the best yields could be obtained from specific sites and localities between about 240 and 300 metres above sea level, in areas in which there was adequate precipitation, which meant that they endured heavy rain every day. In order to obtain sufficient supplies from this needle in a sodden rainforest haystack, they employed the skills and knowledge of the locals and their mules, who could move with ease (but not without accident or contracting diseases like pneumonia and pleurisy) through the impossible terrain.

If Aneurin Bevan ever read the stirring account of the resurrection of this herbal drug in the *National Geographic Magazine*, he certainly didn't understand its implications. The pleas of the National Association of Medical Herbalists and the British Herbal Union to be part of the National Health System fell on deaf ears. The legislators may have missed the point, but not so the pharmaceutical industry. Plant products once more became all the rage, and very soon good pharmacognosists (scientists who knew their materia medica) were in short supply as age-old remedies were hauled out of the undergrowth into the light of modern research and media exposure.

The green hellebore (the plant that must never be taken with mandrake) because of potentially lethal drug interaction) now came under scrutiny once more, and was shown to yield alkaloids effective against high blood pressure. The Swiss giant Ciba-Geigy brought reserpine on to the expanding market in 1954. At first the product was extracted from the Indian snakeroot, as it had been for centuries in the Caribbean where it was used as a sedative and a hyportensive. They soon learned to synthesise it, but only to find that the natural product caused fewer patient problems and was cheaper to produce. Chemists also learned that, although it might be easy to patent a pure synthetic chemical and so recoup the escalating costs of research, development and screening, it was not so easy to patent a plant or the accumulated knowledge of twenty thousand years. And how could you screen all the chemical components of a plant so as to assure yourself, your insurance companies and the public that they were not killing as they were curing? This was an especially important consideration at that time, when new iatrogenic (drug- and lifestyle-induced) syndromes were beginning to fill more and more hospital beds in America and in Europe.

The trouble was that wherever the industry looked within the families of plants, it found a medicine chest overflowing with promise, giving scientific substance to herbal substances that had been in use across the centuries. Africa became a fount of hope. Another liana, this time from the rainforests of Nigeria (what little were left of them), was the highly toxic Calabar bean, *Physostigma venenosum*. This had been used in West Africa and in Madagascar (it is now down to its last 5 per cent of forest) as a trial-by-ordeal poison to determine guilt or innocence (apparently, the victim died if guilty, survived if innocent). This herbal ducking-stool is now a major tool of ophthalmology and is used for the treatment of glaucoma, as the physostigmine it contains produces protracted dilation of the pupil. From Madagascar came also the rosy periwinkle (*Catharanthus roseus*), which became the species *célèbre* of herbal medicine. Researched to the depth it deserved, it was shown to contain vincristine and vinblastine, just two of what look like a whole family of drugs that are in their synthetic form already breathing longer life into 'terminal' cases of childhood leukaemia and Hodgkin's disease. *Strophanthus*, a number of species of which were once used in arrow poisons, provides a source of ouabain, a stimulant still used in cases of acute heart failure and cardiac oedema.

Perhaps the most significant discovery during this period of the ascendancy of plants was that relating to human hormones. With the successful identification and isolation of insulin, the active principle of pancreatic tissue, back in 1923, the search was on for other useful products from slaughterhouse offal. But extraction proved very expensive and commercially almost impossible: for example, it took a tonne of bulls' testicles to provide a paltry 300 milligrams of pure testosterone. Russell E. Marker, a brilliant biochemist, then came to the amazing conclusion that it would be easier to obtain from plants the chemical messengers that control so much of the bodily activity of humans, since plants contain humans' steroidal precursors. Investigation of hundreds of likely species led Marker to the Mexican yam (Dioscorea spp.), and he found that the diosgenin it contained could be chemically converted into the female hormone progesterone which could itself be transformed into its male counterpart testosterone. He knew he had discovered a remarkable stone of biochemical alchemy, but both the world of science and the company for which he worked were incredulous of his claims. So he left for Mexico, where he set up a company called Syntex, which produced the oral contraceptive pill. The rest is herb-based history and, perhaps, one of its most important chapters to date.

No wonder, then, that 1953 saw the founding in Germany of the

Society for Research into Medical Plant Therapy and 1956 the launch of the American Society of Pharmacognosy. Each had its in-house journal, *Planta Medica* and *Lloydia* respectively, to spread the good news of the herbal renaissance. In 1970 *The Atlas of Commonly Used Chinese Traditional Drugs* was published by the Chinese Academy of Sciences, another example of a revival of traditional medicine after years of disrepute. The public, too, were beginning to climb on to the bandwagon of environmental and personal concern: Rachel Carson's book *Silent Spring* sowed very effective seeds of doubt about the chemicals released into the food chain, and pertinent questions began to be asked – not only about pesticides and the likes of the defoliant Agent Orange, but also about food additives and novel drugs like thalidomide.

The changes that have taken place over the past fifty years, with ever more manipulated food, antibiotics and magic salves and cures engineered by ever fewer multinational companies, mean that at least the rich can live a longer active life and, in essence, die without pain. I have never yet met anyone who would like to go back to the bad old days. But the ever spiralling cost of the NHS and problems such as the thalidomide fiasco still in people's minds, the growing fear of 'superbugs', tolerant of all antibiotics, lurking in the corners even of hi-tec hospitals and modern mega-abbatoirs – none of this bodes well for the future. Add to that mad cow disease with prions jumping not over the moon but across genetic barriers, let alone retroviruses punching holes in immune systems, and something has to be done. And something may be. For despite continued political attack against herbal medicine, the big drug companies are spending ever more money on research into ancient herbal remedies. They must surely believe that there is hope of finding at least some cures, which could be double-blind-tested, proved to work, then patented.

The strict botanical definition of a herb is a plant that has no woody parts above ground, thus distinguishing it from shrubs and trees. Any good dictionary then goes on to explain that the word 'herb' has also come to mean a plant (hence including shrubs and trees) used in medicine, and aromatic plants used in cookery. So as you read on through this book you won't be surprised that a number of the healing herbs are woody, even giant trees, and that many of them started their lives as food, flavouring or aperitives. When you take a herbal remedy in its basic form your body is receiving a package deal containing sugars, fats, proteins, trace elements, vitamins and roughage, a package deal tried and tested over thousands of years, not only on animals but on generations of humans as well. Some have been found to be especially effective – say, on the skin or in the stomach – and over the years apothecaries, druggists and chemists have done their best to discover and concentrate their active principles. Sometimes there have been disastrous results, as during the heydays of 'heroic medicine' and, later, of chemotherapeutics.

Tailor-made drugs, in their pure synthesised form, are often a single chemical moiety that is not only new to science but may be new to evolution. The first one was aspirin, although here the chemical company had borrowed the formula from willow bark and meadowsweet, both traditional herbal cures for headaches. Today aspirin is used for thinning the blood and helping to ward off heart attacks (but long-term use can have disastrous effects on the stomach wall).

Like human beings, each plant is an individual and all herbal medicines are characterised by great diversity. In their natural forms, that have been tested over thousands of years, they come as a package deal complete with all the contents of the living cells that made them from sunshine, water and minerals. In contrast, synthetic drugs are very uniform – often a single moiety of a single molecule. Little wonder then that our bodies may react to these new drugs with allergy and even rejection, so they must be handled with even greater care. This was the problem with thalidomide: the molecular twist in the tail of that horrendous story was that one isomer, one mirror image form of the molecule, worked and was safe; unfortunately, it was another that was put on the market.

Also, new chemicals have to be packaged so that the body will accept them. This is of course nothing new: Dr Bach's Flower Remedies – the very popular flower essences on sale in health stores and pharmacies today – are served in alcohol; vitamin supplements come in capsules, many are made of gelatine, the boiled-down dross of the abattoir (not the most reassuring additive for vegetarians, or perhaps for any of us, now that we face the problems of life with mad cows – thank goodness plant-based gelatine substitutes are now available). However, like processed food many of the latest chemicals contain their own protective chemicals – stabilisers (to increase shelf life) and other new additives such as synthetic flavours, fragrances and colours. These are often novel chemicals, brand-new molecules with brand-new names, fighting for space with the brand names on bottles, sprays or pop-out foil.

Thanks in part to the old adage about a spoonful of sugar sweetening the pill, millions of pounds are spent trying to attach a new, 'alien' drug or an engineered antibiotic to a more natural substance, often a sugar – all this in the hope that it will be readily accepted by the virus, the bacterium and the human body, and speed the new chemical on its way to its target enzyme system. Little wonder, then, that since the package deals of many ancient herbal remedies, tried and tested across the ages, contain natural sugars, lipids and proteins, they were readily accepted by the human chemistry and did good wherever they went to work. And the ones that worked their wonders gave their handlers the respect they deserved, as they passed on the heritage of herbal knowledge to future generations, while those that backfired often sent part of that same corpus of knowledge up in flames at the stake, or down with the ducking-stool.

4

The Body Beautiful, or Corporate

Perhaps the dirtiest trick of creative evolution is that there appear to be two types of human beings, Pharaoh's fat and Pharaoh's lean kind. So far, evidence suggests that although this is not genetically controlled, some of us spend our lives dieting while others can carry on eating and always stay trim. But that's the way you are, and you can't rush out and buy a new model as you can with a car. But, like the car, you can keep yourself well serviced and in perfect trim. What is more, it needn't cost you a lot of money: in fact, in a perfect world, it should be cheaper to live the healthy way. The problem is that more and more of us are living in the fast lane without having bothered to read the instruction manual. There may be some excuse for the executive few, grabbing a limp salmon sandwich as they gridlock from fax to boardroom, but for the growing number of couch potatoes we must ask why are we doing it to ourselves. Why fast food? Why all the rush? All it really seems to do is give us more time to take less exercise, while amusing ourselves to death watching fast-food, detergent and car ads, interspersed with soaps about family life and get-rich-quick game shows in which people are paid exorbitant amounts of money to play the games we used to play in the park. We have in fact taken on the executive lifestyle without the pay or the perks. We have even taken on the worry and the stress, because deep down we know that our bank balances can't really afford it. And the sad fact is that neither can our bodies.

Back in the Swinging Sixties, the American government was very worried about the the cost of unnecessary healthcare and time lost in the workplace due to the bad eating habits and the lethargy of the bulk (and again, that is the operative word) of the nation. So concerned were they that their official body, the Food and Nutrition Board of the National Research Council, began to publish, and still publishes, recommended dietary allowances (RDAs), which are updated all the time as research continues.

The seven pillars of Uncle Sam's RDA wisdom
(1) Eat a variety of foods.
(2) Maintain a healthy weight.
(3) Choose a diet low in saturated fat (and that includes cholesterol).
(4) Choose a diet with plenty of vegetables, fruit and grain products.
(5) Use sugars only in moderation.
(6) Use salt or other forms of sodium in moderation.
(7) If you drink alcoholic beverages, do so in moderation.

The Food and Nutrition Board's guidelines are for all normally healthy children and adults, and the reason it gives for its recommendations is to help reduce the risk of heart disease, obesity, high blood pressure, stroke and certain forms of cancer. Unfortunately, like that more recent government health warning seen here in Britain, 'Smoking Kills', many people ignore even the best advice. Forty years on, people on both sides of the Atlantic are still piling on the fat. In Britain almost 1 in 5 people is classified as obese, and in the USA the weight of 1 in 3 reaches danger levels with many more overweight.

GOOD FAT, BAD FAT

Fat is not a cool thing to have. In fact, it never has been, for fat is a good insulator. Whales need a lot of it to keep warm in the cold and salty water, which also helps support their buoyant bulk. We have to stand upright with only thin air to support our bodies, whether fat or thin, and the temperature of the air fluctuates much more than the temperature of the sea. It's one reason why we had to invent clothes, something more comfortable we can slip into whatever the weather. Sadly, it's more difficult to slip off the fat when we get too hot.

What are little girls made of? – sugar and spice and 20–25 per cent fat, which is stored mainly under the skin where it can produce those unsightly lumps and bumps but is always there ready to be called on during pregnancy and lactation. What are little boys made of? – slugs and snails and only 15–20 per cent fat, stored mainly like a camel stores stuff in its hump, but around the belly. You may not like it, but belly fat is very special stuff, for it is used and replaced three times faster than the stuff that gets under our skin. One theory is that belly fat is a rapid-action energy store that helped our ancestors' dads get up and go hunting to supply food for the family. No need to blame the invention of beer, those plasticine bellies have been hanging around since the Pleistocene.

Despite this excuse, statistics from more than twenty countries have put a new twist into the message of this playground joke, for they have proved that being male is seriously bad for your health. At any age, we males are seriously disadvantaged in the survival stakes because the grim reaper has his or her sights on us. The worst period is between twenty and twenty-four, when men are three times more likely to die than women. Being male is now the main cause of early death by any means – from car crash to heart disease and even murder.

Most of the fat we worry about is the bit that shows and makes our bodies crease or sag, and we *should* worry, because it slows us down and makes our hearts and lungs work harder. But fat in the right amount and in the right place does a number of very important jobs, and research is proving that if we had no fat at all we would be in real trouble. For a start, it acts as a shock-absorbing bubble-wrap that protects our internal organs-and pads our heels, fingers and joints – it even lines the sockets of our eyes. If we take a look at fat under a microscope we find that it is not unlike bubble-wrap, for it consists of a honeycomb of big round cells, each one filled with a droplet of fat (our family calls it 'jubble-wrap'). While these sedentary fatty deposits are pretty quiet on the metabolic front, on others they play a far more active role. Served with a network of blood vessels and wired into the nervous system, fat is poised to respond to your body's every energy need.

Certainly the strangest and perhaps the most important thing fat does for us is that it talks to the rest of our body. No, not that gurgling in your tummy – fat is much more subtle than a few slurps and burps. It sits at the heart of a complex and wide-ranging communications network, sending tiny chemical messengers fuelled with a substance called 'leptin' that are carried around in your bloodstream and keep the brain informed of how much energy you have left in your rapid-response fat tanks. If there are a lot of leptin messages in circulation, on go the brakes, we don't feel hungry and we stop eating. If there are too few leptin messages in the pipelines, then alarm bells start ringing as our energy accounts start wandering into overdraft, we get very hungry and rush to the fridge.

But there's much more to leptin than meets the eye: it also helps the body to decide whether it has enough resources to afford the expensive luxuries of adolescence and reproduction, and it plays a crucial role in the protective action of the immune system. In fact, it is a Jack and Jill of all trades, doing everything from balancing your energy books and regulating your fertility, to supplying and commanding your defences against a variety of undesirables. Some scientists think it may even have a say in our mood, behaviour and hormonal responses. So perhaps fat is a pretty cool thing to have as long as it's in the right place and there's not too much of it. I know if you are like me, one of the jubbly kind, it's very hard to say 'no' to that extra helping. It makes my mouth water just thinking about it. But don't give in, fill up on fruit and veg and always take exercise when you can (but never go mad with it, even when you are back on the trim track).

The more we learn about fat, the more fascinating it becomes – so fascinating and so important that scientists are beginning to call it an organ, akin to our liver, pancreas and skin. Fat doesn't just hang around and get in the way of a healthy life, it is part of the system that controls that healthy life. Too much fat is perhaps the first symptom of a disease that is now debilitating the rich world, and today warnings are rife that parents may live longer than their couch-potato offspring.

As I type, reports come through that up to one-third of all fat people are infected with adenovirus 36, the kind of virus that is responsible for colds, diarrhoea and conjunctivitis and – wait for it – obesity in animals. Animals have six times the normal level of adenovirus-36 infection found in people without weight problems. So perhaps it is possible to catch fat – if so, roll on the roll-off cure. Even that might be at hand, thanks to the Kalahari Bushmen, descendants of Eve, some of whom still live as their forefathers did not far from the mother lode of humanity.

HOODIA CACTUS
Hoodia gordoni

AFRICA

If you live in a desert, the search for food not only keeps you fit and on the move, it occupies much of your working day. The Bushmen of the Kalahari include in their diet a prickly plant, erroneously called the Hoodia cactus. The error in this English name comes from the fact that no true cacti grow naturally in the Old World. *Hoodia gordoni*, which is a member of the milkweed family and a succulent, can be found growing in abundance in times of drought. The Bushmen must originally have chewed it to ward off the pangs of hunger, and discovered that it did just that.

Sadly, the end of the last millennium put a new twist in the tale of this potential fat-buster. The Bushmen of the Kalahari had long been the subject of intensive study by anthropologists and their kin. At some point the facts about the Hoodia were passed on to the South African Council for Scientific and Industrial Research, which evidently isolated the active ingredient, then patented it as 'P57' before liaising with a British firm which dreamed up the following unique double-blind test. Nineteen fat people were locked in a house for two weeks and were offered three unlimited meals a day and access to snacks in between. Those taking a placebo ate 3,200 calories a day, while those taking P57 ate only 2,200 (the usual average is 2,800 for an active male).

On the basis of its research, the firm sold the patent on for the not unprincely sum of many millions. The only trouble was that no one had told the Bushmen about it. Litigation is already under way, backed by a group who helped argue the Bushmen's case in 1999 when they were given back rights of ownership to 100,000 hectares of farmland on the edge of the Namibian Desert.

When is a food not a food? When it's been proved that it's a drug that can relieve pain, promote health or prolong our active lives – it's patently obvious. Watch this space, for the ultimate of slimming pills could be on the market within three years.

TOMATO
Lycopersicun esculentum

When first introduced into Europe in Elizabethan times, tomatoes were thought to have aphrodisiac properties and so were sold under the name of 'love apples'. More recently the high consumption of tomatoes was said to be linked to a high incidence of cancer in the population. As with the aphrodisiacal claims, no link with cancer was ever proven beyond the suggestion that the ketchup culture goes hand in hand with a high intake of saturated fat. Indeed, according to Harvard Medical School, Boston, a survey of the most recent research (1986–98) confirms that frequent consumption of tomato products is associated with a lower risk of prostate cancer. Research suggests that lycopene, the natural pigment that gives tomatoes and watermelons their colour, is the active principle, and that levels of this dietary antioxidant vary greatly in tomato-containing products. Lycopene is known to destroy cancer cells and to restore the gaps between those cells which, unchecked, allow cancers to proliferate.

It has also been shown, Europe-wide, that when ingested in its natural food form lycopene increases the oxidation resistance of low-density lipids (LDL). Along with other powerful antioxidants lycopene shows promise as a biomarker that might be used to help define the optimal diets for humans. This gift from the New World is good news indeed, but be selective: take a look on the juice carton or the ketchup bottle to see what food-processing it has endured – and beware GM tomatoes, square or round.

GRAIN AMARANTHS
Amaranthus spp.

Made illegal by the conquistadors' missionaries on grounds of association with bloody sacrifice, the grain amaranths once produced the bulk of the flour used by Aztec royalty and the peoples of the High Andes. They are not cereals but are related to the garden flower love-lies-bleeding. Known for two thousand years and described by Pliny the Elder, amaranths are edible and medicinal plants comprising many species, some of which are best known in the West as colourful pot plants and garden summer annuals rather than as food or medicine. Christians adorned their saints with amaranth, and the plants still have an important role in Vanuatuan (South Pacific) ceremonies as they did in Aztec culture.

As many people are today becoming allergic to cereals, making it very difficult for them to plan a healthful diet, bread, cakes and biscuits made from the flour of the grain amaranths are coming into their own. Young leaves and old, even non-woody stalks, are becoming haute cuisine in America, used instead of spinach in various dishes and as a highly colourful garnish. With a higher protein content than cereals, amaranths are also high in fibre, lysine and other essential amino acids, as well as vitamins and minerals including iron, and so are great news for everyone. Most recent research suggests amaranth oil as an alternative to that derived from marine animals as a natural source of squalene, which chemically resembles sebum, making it useful in skin-moisturising products and as a herbal alternative to the immunity-system-boosters said to be derived from the livers of sharks.

CABBAGE
Brassica oleracea var. capitata
MEDITERRANEAN

Cabbage juice is a traditional remedy in northern European countries, having been valued for its healing properties since the time of Christ. It has been used for stomach ache, ulcers, poor digestion, bronchitis, coughs and rheumatic symptoms.

In more recent times, a cabbage-soup diet has been used in hospitals in both the USA and the UK as part of a pre-operative weight-loss regime. It is a serious medicinal diet to be used for about two weeks, and is mostly employed to quickly dispense with internal fatty tissue that may complicate operations such as those dealing with gall bladder or gallstones. Thus is the medical profile of the humble cabbage elevated. Sadly, though, it is not a quick fix, as weight will slowly reassert itself if a poor diet is maintained or a better one is not established post-operatively. Research also suggests that eating both cabbage and nuts during pregnancy can help protect babies from allergies, and that the vitamin E in both foods helps guard against degenerative brain disease. So eating up your greens may well be a brainy thing to do.

TAMARIND
Tamarindus indica
AFRICA

Tamarindus is derived from the Arabic *tamr-Hindi*, 'date of India'. It is an integral part of many recipes from South-East Asia. Tamarind originates from Africa and migrated with the Spanish to the West Indies and Mexico in the seventeenth century. It is a sweet and sour, astringent, stimulant herb that is used to improve digestion. It incorporates antiseptic and laxative effects and can be drunk as a herb tea. The sweetish acidic fruit is also an ingredient in cardiac and blood-sugar-reducing medicine.

In Ayurvedic medicine, tamarind is used to improve the appetite, strengthen the stomach and relieve constipation, and when mixed with cumin and sugar as a treatment for dysentery. The low incidence of kidney-stones in the Indonesian population that uses Ayurvedic medicine has been attributed to the frequent inclusion of tamarind in the diet. It is deduced that the tartrates in the rind of the fruit inhibit the formation of calcium oxalate stones by decreasing the amount of ionised calcium in the urine.

In Chinese medicine, tamarind is considered a 'cooling herb' and used as a febrifuge to treat summer overheating. The fruit is also eaten for loss of appetite, nausea and vomiting in pregnancy. Tamarind's hydroxycitric acid content helps to inhibit the conversion of carbohydrates into fats, regulates the conversion by the liver of excess glucose into stored fats and cholesterol, and helps maintain healthy overall levels of fat in the blood. It also reduces feelings of hunger and increases energy and fat metabolism. Research has demonstrated that a polysaccharide of tamarind can modulate the immune system.

Tamarind should not be taken with aspirin or other pain-relievers, as it enhances their effects and may produce adverse reactions and side-effects.

SWEET FENNEL
Foeniculum vulgare
MEDITERRANEAN

Not to be confused with bitter fennel, sweet fennel is thought to have originated in Malta and spread via the monks who included it in their medicinal repertoire during the wars of the Crusades. The plant grown for oil is today cultivated in France, Italy, Greece and Hungary. The oil is anti-inflammatory, antiseptic and antimicrobial with carminative effects. It induces or assists menstruation, increases the secretion of milk in lactation, and is an expectorant and laxative. Sweet fennel acts on the spleen, and is a digestive aid and tonic that can alleviate poor appetite. The oil's ability to counter obesity lies in its diuretic and detoxifying effects which help combat impurity in the blood and organs. It also stimulates the circulation and so carries its good effects throughout the body. Italian research has found the oil to be highly antioxidant, comparable in some cases to vitamin C, and antimicrobial, attacking many forms of plant and animal bacteria. It is relatively non-toxic, but narcotic in large doses.

As psychotropic medication has been shown to pose major health risks in children treated for ADHD (Attention Deficit Hyperactivity Disorder), the medical profession has been researching different diets and supplements of vitamins, minerals and sedative herbs for these patients. Fennel is among those herbal aids that promise to be of use.

SUNFLOWER
Helianthus annuus
NEW WORLD

The Aztecs worshipped the sun, and they and many other groups of America's native people selected sunflower plants from the wild and developed them into the fantastic crop they are today. *The Guinness Book of Records* tells us that the world's tallest has topped 7.76 metres, while all good herbal books, and parrots, sing the praises of the seeds and the oil extracted from them, which is rich in polyunsaturated fatty acids.

The essentially odourless oil of this nutritious herb contains vitamins A, D and E in particular, with good supplies of mineral calcium, zinc, potassium, iron and phosphorus. The raw buds and seed sprouts can be added to salads, and the buds are also steamed as a vegetable. Culinary use of the oil helps lower blood cholesterol levels and soothe irritated tissues. The unrefined oil should not be used in cooking at high temperatures, as it breaks down and produces toxic elements when heated. The unrefined, unblended oil has a softening and moisturising effect on the skin and is used for massage; organic sunflower oil is often used as a maceration base for other healing herbs. Research has shown that sunflower oil in the diet might also be helpful in the treatment of multiple sclerosis, and that the naturally occurring fatty acid CLA can be derived from sunflowers. CLA has been identified as a potentially key factor in weight management and is the key ingredient in a number of new weight-loss preparations. The oil can also be burned in lamps.

ALFALAFA
Medicago sativa
ASIA, CHINA

Alfalfa has been used for digestive problems in Chinese and Indian medicine for thousands of years. It gained popularity in the West recently for its apparent cholesterol-lowering property.

The plant is a good source of vitamins A, B_1, B_6, C, E and K, as well as calcium, potassium, iron and zinc. The alfalfa leaf poses no problems when used as a herb at customary dosage levels.

Discovery of an oestrogen-like action in animal tests has led to its use as a remedy for the symptoms of the menopause. Although alfalfa has been used as a treatment for diabetes, thyroid conditions, arthritis and water retention, until recently only its effect on appetite has been verified. Russian animal research has now found that the luceron it contains stimulates the secretion of bile and normalises the synthesis of bile acids; hence it may be of use against hepatitis. Earlier Irish research of *Medicago*'s traditional anti-diabetic effects (in mice) also shows scientific promise. In North America, alfalfa's calcium content, as well as that of oat straw and horsetail, is traditionally effective in the long-term treatment of osteoporosis.

Avoid the sprouts if you have SLE (systemic lupus erythematosus) or if you suffer from an auto-immune disease.

AUBERGINE
Solanum melongena

ASIA, INDIA

Aubergine is today a main garden crop in Mediterranean countries and in subtropical areas, and its fruits are commonly referred to as 'eggs'. The fruit helps lower blood cholesterol levels and, like many other non-fattening vegetables, makes an excellent constituent of an anti-cholesterol diet.

Research has proved that the aubergine's flavonoids, and nasunin, an anthocyanin, have potent antioxidant effects. The fruit has been used raw as a poultice for haemorrhoids but is usually made into an ointment for this purpose. Both the fruit and its juice are diuretic, and the leaves when pulped make a cooling paste for treating burns and other skin lesions. Please do not use as a home remedy, because the preparation must be done by experts. Aubergine leaves are toxic and can only be applied externally.

BELL PEPPER
Capsicum annuum var. annuum
SOUTH AMERICA

This tropical treasure, varieties of which grow readily in the Mediterranean, is a powerhouse of antioxidants, vitamin C and carotenes. Ripe sweet peppers vary in colour from red through orange and yellow to green, and all have similar properties, but the orange and red ones contain more antioxidant anthocyanins and beta-carotene. Red peppers contain one of the highest concentrations of antioxidants found in everyday food. These help prevent heart disease, cancer, stroke and cataracts. A raw red pepper holds more than 100mg of vitamin C (more than half the daily requirement), the optimum one could expect from a single food. The high levels of beta-carotenes that convert to vitamin A ensure a sound supply of body armour. The sweet pepper contains bioflavonoids, which have strong antioxidant properties and are thought to help prevent certain kinds of cancer.

The latest research and the discovery of new glycosides strengthen the claims for the importance of the sweet pepper in the Mediterranean diet. As a herb the red pepper is an enormous boon to the immune system. The common or garden sweet pepper, not being 'hot', is not of the variety that contains large amounts of capsaicin, which is the main therapeutic and flavouring compound in cayenne and antimicrobial chilli peppers. Both sweet and chilli peppers well deserve the name 'food medicine' for their antioxidant potential alone.

PAWPAW, PAPAYA
Carica papaya
SOUTH AMERICA

Found in the tropical forests of South America, the fragrant fruit is now grown in similar climates around the world. The sweet and juicy papaya fruit is very nutritious and a good source of beta-carotene and vitamin C, helping to prevent damage from free radicals. Half a small pear-shaped fruit can provide the adult RDA of vitamin C, plus calcium and iron. The fruit and its juice, containing papain, an enzyme similar to pepsin produced by the human digestive system to break down proteins, are mainly employed for digestive disorders and in the food industry as a tenderiser. Papain is used externally in ointments prescribed for the treatment of severe wounds or slow-healing wounds and ulcers, helping to dissolve dead tissue without damaging living cells. Papain also exhibits pain-relieving properties, and is approved by the American Food and Drug Administration (FDA) for use in spinal injections to ease the discomfort of slipped discs.

In the commercial world papain is used in the manufacture of chewing-gum, in the clarification of beer, termite control, and the shrink-proofing of wool and silk. There is exciting ongoing research into the scientific basis for the traditional use of papaya fruits and leaves as a malaria remedy in parts of Africa and India.

As a food medicine, papaya fruits are safe to eat, except in certain medical and pregnancy conditions where there is a bleeding disorder that its extracts could aggravate. There is some evidence of allergic reactions.

BROCCOLI
Brassica spp.
MEDITERRANEAN

Broccoli probably originated somewhere in Turkey, where much of the selection and the first steps in the breeding of cabbages and other members of the cabbage flower family took place. Arriving in Tuscany during the eighth century BC, it became very popular in Rome where the calabrese variety was widely used, and reached Britain in the eighteenth century. Thomas Jefferson, farmer and statesman, showed his independence by planting it in his garden near Charlottesville on 27 May 1767. It was finally brought into popularity in America by the d'Arrigo brothers, immigrants from Messina, who back in the 1930s ran a thriving broccoli business that even sponsored a radio programme complete with adverts. Sadly, they didn't call it 'New Broccoli', perhaps for fear of litigation from 'Grand Old Opry'.

Long considered one of the crown jewels of nutrition – and so it should be, because in fact you are eating the whole flowerhead, packed full of all the goodness needed to produce the plant's flowers, fruits and seeds – broccoli is a great source of vitamins A, B_1, B_2, B_3, B_6, C and E, calcium, iron, magnesium, potassium and zinc, and useful trace minerals. Eat it cooked or raw, but always remember that boiling can remove much of its goodness.

Research at the Johns Hopkins Medical School in America found that sulforaphane glucosinolate (SGS), a natural antioxidant constituent of broccoli and other members of the cabbage flower family, blocked the formation of mammary tumours in rats. On the basis of these findings a Brassica Chemoprotection Laboratory was set up in the university. Among other things this led to the development of patented BrocoSprouts, 30g of which contain as much SGS as 550g of cooked (not boiled) mature broccoli. Epidemiological evidence suggests that eating that much broccoli every week provides significant health benefits.

5

Skin Deep – and a Nice Head of Hair

YOUR LARGEST ORGAN

How deep *is* your skin? Well, it depends on where you measure it. In places like the soles of your feet where it is subject to wear and tear, it is much thicker than elsewhere. Skin is the largest organ of your body and your first line of defence. It helps keep pathogenic organisms out and water and salt under control, and it does its best to protect you from chemical and physical damage. What is more, it comes punctured with three million sweat glands and loses forty thousand skin flakes, the equivalent of forty million dead cells, every day. No wonder that under normal conditions skin heals very quickly, and thank goodness for those millions of house-dust mites that gorge themselves on the stuff and so keep our beds and houses clean.

Lesions, wounds or trauma click a whole chain of complex bio-chemical events into action. The wounded tissue releases the hormone thromboplastin, which converts prothrombin into thrombin. That converts water-soluble fibrinogen into waterproof fibrin which forms a mesh, trapping red corpuscles and thus stemming the flow of blood. The fibrin mesh slowly contracts, squeezing out plasma as the scab forms. Clever old you – you do all that every time you nick yourself with the razor. (A scab on the outside is OK, but when the same sequence of chemical changes happens within your bloodstream, thrombosis looms.)

Your skin's outer layer, or epidermis, contains its own self-adjust-ing sunblock called 'melanin'; that's why we tan. But please take it extra-easy when you're in the sun, because whether you believe in ozone holes or not, even those with the blackest skins can scorch after a winter in the shade. Although carotenes *may* help reduce the risk of developing skin cancer, sunscreens are now a must. The choice is enormous and many are well researched – none more so than adequate clothing. The epidermis also produces a waterproofing agent called 'keratin' and, being well supplied with breathing pores, this is Gore-Tex in living guise.

Proteins such as keratin and collagen give strength and elasticity not only to the skin, but to hair and tendons as well. Collagen is the intercellular material that binds cells together and is found in skin, ligaments, bone and cartilage. It is a very tough material, with a strength equal to that of high-tensile steel. It is rich in the non-essential amino acids glycine, proline and hydroxyproline. It accounts for about 30 per cent of all the protein in humans and each molecule is made up of three thousand amino acids, which are evenly distributed in three intertwined, cross-linked chains that provide significant structural rigidity. Thank goodness our bodies can make these bulk amino acids – if they couldn't, we would soon get an attack of the sags.

Below the epidermis is the dermis, a tough, flexible layer made mostly of connective tissue with lots of nerves and blood vessels, lymphatic and fat cells. The latter are for insulation and protection, the former to keep the whole thing – sorry, you – in touch with the world outside, alive and able to blush.

Sweat glands, all three million of them, not only allow you to sweat at least eight litres a day and so keep cool by water evaporation, but also help regulate salt balance and get rid of waste and other unwanted substances. The sweat glands are backed up by the sebaceous glands, which produce an oily secretion important in conditioning our hair, including our finest silky hairs on our foreheads, alongside the nose, down the centre of the chest and around the anus. The rest appear to make us smell as we humans should smell. The question of whether these self-made fragrances are social or sexual, helping to control our lifestyles or our sex drive, is still a subject of fragrant research.

Itching, like blushing, is the first sign of trouble ahead, so find out what's wrong and cure it. Don't scratch about playing with the symptoms; you may only make them worse. Dermatitis is an inflammation of the skin, causing a rash. Substances to which you are allergic often act as a trigger. The most infamous case is that of the little boy in

America who, experiencing no allergy himself, picked a bunch of wild flowers containing poison ivy for his teacher. Sadly, she died. Many people today are allergic or develop allergies to certain combinations of chemicals like detergent. The cure is to find out what's causing it and stay away from that substance completely. Allergies to dairy products and cereals are becoming commoner, and exactly why this is so is still a matter of debate. Anyway, a radical change in the diet of the afflicted individuals is called for.

The most important thing of all for skin care, from both the inside and out, is simply water. Contrary to what is often thought, skins of whatever type suffer not from lack of oil but from lack of water. Modern living, with central heating, air conditioning and the like, makes the situation worse. Drinks made with water and additives are not enough – pure, cleansing water is what the body needs, inside and out. Fruits and vegetables contain proteins, fats and carbohydrates in plenty, and each one is also a reservoir of water there for the taking. Water hydrates the skin. What is more, it comes complete with a *soupçon* of all the minerals needed to keep both plants and us healthy.

While on the subject of minerals, selenium, mentioned earlier, is important to skin as it is a key component in the making of all protective cell membranes. As with all other minerals, selenium levels in food are related to their presence in the soil. New Zealand's soils are so low in selenium that dietary deficiencies are common. In the USA levels are in many places not much better, while in parts of China keshan disease caused by selenium deficiency is endemic, and children may die of heart failure. Fortunately, selenium is found in citrus fruits, avocado pears and whole grains, as well as in offal, meats, fish and shellfish, and dairy produce (especially butter).

The primary requirement for a healthy skin is not just a 'balanced diet' containing a decent supply of vitamins, minerals and fatty acids, but proper management of this your largest organ and your first line of environmental protection. The importance of vitamin C as well as vitamin E in the skin-repair tool-kit lies in their antioxidant and nutrient value, not to mention their basic role in the production of face-lifting collagen and connective tissue that endow the owner with a soft, smooth skin. B vitamins are also important to skin; and beta-carotene, a precursor of vitamin A, helps the growth and repair of body tissues and plays a part in maintaining the skin's well-being.

Plenty of water, physical exercise and a daily allowance of fresh air are of crucial importance. Fresh air usually comes with exposure to sunshine, and our skin has the ability to process sunshine to make vitamin D (calciferol). Elderly and house- and office-bound people are inclined not to get enough sunshine or water, which can cause skin problems to arise. Vitamin D is essential for calcium and phosphate control and for bone formation.

Alpha-hydroxyacids (AHAs) are naturally occurring acids found in fruits and other foods that help to keep the skin in good health. For instance, citric acid is derived from citrus fruits such as oranges, and glycolic acid comes from sugar cane. Alpha-hydroxyacids have been used for many centuries, Cleopatra being their most famous advocate. As found in our foods, they are safe when used in cosmetics in low concentrations and, unlike chemical peels, alpha-hydroxyacid peels are not toxic to the skin.

Although Cleopatra is fabled for bathing in ass's milk to cleanse her skin and so enhance her beauty, goat's milk was used on a more modest scale as a facial cleansing agent by the ancient Celts. Science is only now catching up with the knowledge of the ancients, and today's cosmetics and toiletries are being improved by the use of natural phytochemicals, in the form of botanical extracts. Clearly, the wily Egyptians and Celts could not formally analyse their choice of milk as a cleanser, purifier and preservative of the skin, but they certainly knew what they were doing. Wellfed nanny's milk contains fine fats, vitamins B_1, B_2, B_3, B_6, B_{12}, C, D_1, E and folic acid; lactose, casein, chlorine, phosphorus, iodine, iron, sulphur (which attacks the diseases of the skin), zinc, cobalt, arachidic acid, magnesium, potassium, calcium, sodium, copper and gold. No manufactured product comes close to providing so many elements in harmony with the human body and its fundamental requirements. A pad of organic cotton wool and some goat's milk to remove cosmetics provides an unsurpassable daily skin treatment.

OATS

Avena sativa

EUROPE

Avena fatua, 'wild oats', are found in Eurasia and North Africa. A southern European species, they reached northern parts during the Iron Age and became the subsistence crop of Scotland. Cultivated oats (*Avena sativa*), those we eat today, are mostly grown in northern temperate regions, as they need water and humidity and dislike dry weather in early summer.

Oats are so 'everyday' that it takes an old saying such as 'He's feeling his oats' to remind us how stimulating and energising they are. Best known as a nutritious cereal, they are universally recognised as a good daily foundation against seasonal complaints such as winter flu, especially for growing children and the vulnerable elderly. Oat preparations are still taken internally as a remedy for a very broad spectrum of ill health, from digestive problems to heart disease.

Research has shown that oats lower cholesterol, combat the overproduction of prostaglandins (hormones that act on the blood vessels and other organs of the body) and improve stamina. They are considered mildly antidepressant, they stimulate the central nervous system and, by raising energy levels, they help to maintain nervous and physical ability and to bolster the immune system. In the case of athletes, research has proved that oats may help maintain muscle function during training and exercise via their antioxidant activity and by stimulating muscular contraction. Research is under way regarding oats as a preventive for colon cancer, and oat-bran as a way to improve the long-term control of diabetes. They are also beneficial for the prevention of constipation after operations, decreasing the need for purgatives and enemas.

Their use as an emollient for various skin problems is widely accepted. In the developed world eczema affects one baby in ten. The symptoms are broken nights for all concerned, thanks to itching, blistering and scaling skin. The exact causes are not known, and instant cures are unknown. However, having suffered with two of my own children, I can recommend trying porridge oats. A muslin bagful suspended under the hot tap when filling the bath did wonders for our family relationships. But have a care, because more people are becoming allergic to cereals, including porridge. Another good tip learned from experience is to avoid bath additives, even cutting down on bathing if necessary, and babygrows are very good to prevent scratching, which often sets the whole thing off again.

Acne, a disease of the hair follicles and oil-secreting glands, is apparently triggered by the first flush of male hormones and is hence the curse of teenage years just when they want to look their best. Acne conglobata is a more severe form that leads to cyst formation and may leave permanent scars on face, shoulders, torso – and ego. Excess washing, cosmetics, machine oil and scratching should be avoided. And it's well worth trying oats – most likely, you won't be one of the allergic few.

TEA TREE
Melaleuca alternifolia
AUSTRALIA

Native to Australia, mainly New South Wales, the oil of the tea tree is a national treasure and is not produced outside of Australia, where Aborigines have been using it since dreamtime. It got its name from its local usage as a herbal tea prepared from the leaves, and is now one of the most important natural anti-septics used across the world. Good for oily skin, the oil is excellent for healing abscesses, acne, athlete's foot, blisters, burns, herpes (cold sores), dandruff, insect bites, rashes including nappy rash, spots, verrucae, warts and infected wounds, and it has the ability to kill 'nits' (the eggs of head lice). Although several different species are used medicinally by the Aborigines of the northern regions of Australia, the one that has gained acclaim and popularity in the West is *M. alternifolia*.

Tea tree's therapeutic properties were first researched in the 1920s, but it didn't reach Western awareness until used by

Australian forces in the Second World War for dressing wounds. Sadly, from then on it received little further attention until the 1960s. Then the therapeutic cat was let out of the tea-tree bag, for research found that the oil is vigorously active against all three varieties of infectious agents — that is bacteria, viruses and fungi. Recent research suggests that with its lipophilic (fat-loving) nature, which enables it to penetrate the skin, the oil may be suitable for topical therapeutic use in the treatment of fungal, mucosal and cutaneous infections and against yeasts such as candida. The latter inhabit the vagina and alimentary tract and, under certain conditions, cause candidiasis, often in the form of thrush (oral and vaginal). Infection may spread throughout the body, sometimes developing in patients receiving broad-spectrum antibiotics.

Tea tree oil is also a powerful immuno-stimulant, not only killing virulent infections but helping the body to respond to their effects. Melaleuca oils are analgesic to differing degrees. The antiseptic component is well tolerated by the skin; however, the oil also contains varying amounts of cineol, which can irritate. Any allergy is usually mild and transient; allergic-contact dermatitis is probably due to the component eucalyptol present in tea tree oil, so it should be avoided by those with that particular susceptibility.

ALOE
Aloe vera syn. *A. barbadensis*
SOUTHERN AFRICA, MADAGASCAR

Perhaps this plant should be renamed *aloe anita*, because it was Anita Roddick's Body Shop that successfully advertised its virtues to the world.

One of the herbs of the Bible, it has been used to heal burns from time immemorial. Early research in the 1930s in the USA and Russia demonstrated aloe gel's potential for healing wounds, ulcers and burns. The gel puts a protective layer on an affected area and speeds up healing, an action that is partly due to aloectin B, which helps stimulate the immune system. In the 1990s *Aloe barbadensis* gel extract was found to counteract UV-induced suppression of the immune system by a mechanism that does not involve DNA damage. The extract has also been shown to alleviate adult bronchial asthma. Most recent research confirms that a new aloe vera polysaccharide, aloeride, stimulates the immune system, and although it comprises only 0.015 per cent of the aloe juice dry weight, it is alone responsible for the effectiveness of the crude juice. A report in *Clinical Review* in 1987 shows that a compound called acemannon which is found in aloe vera seems to have remarkable antiviral properties, even where the HIV virus is concerned.

Dr Reg McDaniel stated: 'It appears that Carrisyn [a commercial name for acemannon patented by Carrington Laboratories] neutralizes the AIDs virus by transforming its protein envelope thus preventing it from attaching itself to the T4 cells.' Aloe vera research may also prove beneficial in the prevention of some forms of cancer.

The fresh aloe vera plant's wonderfuly soothing leaf 'gel' is easily grown as a kitchen windowsill plant or on a patio for immediate domestic use. Cleopatra regarded the gel as the fountain of youth, and today it ranks among the best skin moisturisers. Aloe gel accelerates the formation of fibroblasts, which help in the manufacture of collagen, the protein that controls the ageing process of the skin. It is also highly moisturising, and is absorbed by the outer layer of the skin three or four times more quickly than water. Recent research shows that it can speed healing after certain forms of cosmetic surgery.

Aloe gel has also been used for wounds, scalds, burns, sunburn, frostbite, eczema and the juice, 'bitter aloes', as a nail-paint to prevent biting. The bactericidal juice is effective against herpes simplex viruses.

Aloe is also used in Ayurvedic medicine as a tonic, a purgative and a rejuvenator. The Russians use it as an antiseptic emollient and laxative, a purgative, a moisturiser and a wound-healer. Used externally, aloe does not appear to pose any problems. However, it should not be used internally for more than a fortnight without consulting a doctor, as it can lead from simple to serious potassium deficiency. Neither should it be taken in pregnancy or by those suffering from irritable bowel syndrome or haemorrhoids. The same is true for those receiving prescribed cardiac glycosides, thiazide diuretics or using corticosteroids or topical or internal hydrocortisone-containing medications. Although the pulp of aloe vera leaves devoid of the gel could be useful in the treatment of non-insulin-dependent diabetes mellitus, the diabetic drug Glyburide should not be taken without first consulting your healthcare practitioner.

The herb would seem to have a lot of as yet untapped healing potential.

AVOCADO
Persea americana
NEW WORLD

Avocados grow on avocado, not pear trees. They are related to magnolia and bay laurel, and are to be found in the swamplands of Mexico, Florida and California, where they got their nickname 'alligator pear'. The Aztecs considered the pure oil extracted from the fruit's flesh an aphrodisiac, and other cultures used it medicinally. Probably the first oil to be cold-pressed, it is highly prized in Central America for cooking. The natural unbleached 'green' oil contains vitamins, A, B_1, B_2 and D, the minerals potassium, phosphorus, magnesium, sulphur, calcium, sodium and copper. Avocado oil is a superb emollient, useful for severely dehydrated skins. Recent research has also found that a vitamin B_{12} cream containing avocado oil has considerable potential as a well tolerated, long-term topical therapy for psoriasis. When taken internally as fruit pulp or capsules, it seems to trigger DNA into producing soluble collagen, which constitutes about 70 per cent of the dermis. This could account for the avocado's moisturising, softening and anti-wrinkle effects, helping to prevent premature ageing. Those who eat the antioxidant avocado can expect a reduction in blood LDLs. Recent research on one of the compounds extracted from the fruit indicates that it might prevent inflammation-associated diseases including cancer. Belgian research has found that other substances present in the avocado (and the soya bean) can alleviate osteoarthritis of the knee. Furthermore, the intake of analgesics decreased by more than 50 per cent in 71 per cent of the same research group, which makes avocado and its oil desirable in the diet of all those affected by osteoarthritis.

It's clear that this fruit is going anything but pear-shaped when it comes to its potential medicinal use.

ROSE OIL
Rosa spp.
EUROPE, ASIA

There are more than ten thousand types of cultivated rose, selected and bred across the millennia. In the main, the choice of medicinal rose depends on the country of origin. Red rose or 'apothecary's rose' (*R. gallica*) oil is traditional in Western medicine; the oriental or tea rose (*R. indica*) is used in Ayurvedic medicine, and the Chinese or Japanese rose (*R. rugosa*) is used in Chinese medicine. Surgeon Ambroise Paré (1510–90) used rose oil topically with great success on traumatic post-operative wounds in the battlefield. Today rose oil's anti-HIV action and that of its pure compounds (*R. damascena*) may be of more current scientific interest, but the rose is an unsurpassable healer of skin. Rosehip oil of the Chilean *rosa mosqueta* (*R. rubiginosa*) is currently renowned for healing post-surgical wounds, ulcerations and scar tissue.

Non-toxic, non-irritant and non-sensitising rose oil, used as a skincare remedy, alleviates dry skin, eczema and herpes, and is kind to sensitive complexions and mature, ageing skin and wrinkles. Astringent rosewater assists with broken capillaries, and it is used as a natural remedial lotion for sensitive and sore eyes and skin, as well as being used culinarily. Rose oil used in aromatherapeutic massage can assist poor circulation and palpitations, such as those experienced by women during the menopause. It has been used for coughs, hay fever and asthma, cholecystitis (inflammation of the gall bladder), liver congestion and nausea. It has had some success in cases of insomnia and headache brought about by nervous tension, and is useful for stress-related complaints generally. Rose oil should not be used internally.

The repertoire of the rose is not yet fully documented. More than six hundred compounds are present in its oil and many are still unidentified. One we do know about is phenylethylamine (PEA), found in rosewater and said to be aphrodisiac, and which is also the 'aphrodisiac' element in chocolate. For those wartime children who were brought up on rosehip syrup, none of this will come as a surprise, especially as we now know that the hips are chock-full of anticarcinogenic anthocyanins and provitamin A (the forerunner of carotenes), which helps to maintain the general health of all our cells.

Red roses for a blue lady — roses are a true gift of Nature for a modern world in need of its antidepressive effects.

ELDERFLOWER
Sambucus nigra
EUROPE

The elder grows in moist, warm temperate climates and in subtropical forests too. In northern Europe it is often found in damp, dark, well manured corners of fields and farmyards. Said to be the tree from which Judas Iscariot hanged himself, in Europe it is also part of folklore tradition, where it has often been called the 'people's medicine chest'. In Russian folk dermatology elderflower infusions are used as an antiseptic wash for skin problems, including chronic eczema, psoriasis, seborrhoea, dermatitis and hair loss. One of the ancient Myddfai treatments (see p. 62) for shingles uses an extract of elder bark.

Elderflower water, or *aqua sambuci*, is skin-freshening and -softening. Used as a wash or compress, an infusion of the bitter, pungent, cooling herb reduces inflammation and soothes irritated skin, and it may be used for mouth ulcers and externally for minor injuries. The active anti-inflammatory principle is thought to be ursolic acid, and it is known that the flowers do reduce inflammation. They are used in skin lotions, creams and ointments, and flower extracts are used topically to help reduce inflammation around muscles and joints. Dr Hauschka, whose holistic products are fêted by celebrities seeking beauty inside and out, recommends elderflower elixir for autumn and winter use to stimulate the elimination of toxins.

The adventurous can lightly fry the flower-heads for breakfast or macerate them in a light carrier oil for massage purposes. Whether as a food medicine or a drink, there are few plants worldwide that give so much free medicinal help and wholesome culinary pleasure.

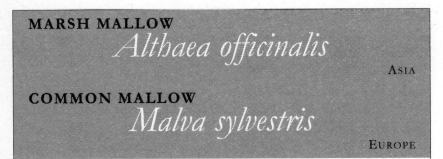

MARSH MALLOW
Althaea officinalis
ASIA

COMMON MALLOW
Malva sylvestris
EUROPE

Although the marsh mallow plant stems from central Asia, it spread rapidly westward to Europe and eastward to China and has been known in Britain since the Roman occupation. Its other English name, 'mortification root', relates to its anti-infection properties, especially those to do with its therapeutic effects on gangrene ('mortification'). In folk medicine, marsh mallow is used as a remedy for burns, constipation, diarrhoea and infected wounds. The Bedouin employ its decoctions externally to soothe inflamed skin. Therapeutically, both leaves and root may be used externally as a soothing poultice and ointment to promote healing, and marsh mallow continues to be used in Western proprietary products in the form of liquid extracts (from the leaves and root), syrup, stomach tablets, tonsillitis mixture and, combined with slippery elm (see p. 199), as a drawing ointment for boils. The mucilages of the plant stimulate the immune system and the production of white blood cells, slow the production of mucus and reduce sugar levels in the body.

Once used in a sweetmeat called *pâté de guimauve*, the common mallow is not as strong as its cousin the marsh mallow. Its leaves and shoots, which have been used as a medicinal pottage herb since the eighth century BC, are both soothing to the gut and laxative, and they continue to be eaten in salads. Like the marsh mallow it is an effective demulcent and the flowers and leaves are emollient. Applied to sensitive areas of the skin or used as a poultice for abscesses or boils it will reduce swelling and draw out toxins, and is also useful for insect bites and weeping eczema.

GRAPEFRUIT
Citrus x paradisi
PACIFIC, POLYNESIA

The dietary importance of oranges, lemons and all the other citrus fruits that have been discovered, selected and bred across the years cannot be overestimated. Although consisting of mainly water, they are a rich source of vitamins B, E and especially C whether eaten raw, juiced or canned, and they have long been used for marmalades.

The grapefruit is an evergreen tree, also called 'shaddock'. It is not known in a wild state, but is thought to have developed as a hybrid in the Caribbean. It is today widely grown for its fruit and its oil, which is used as a fragrance in soaps, detergents, cosmetics and perfumes and as a flavouring for desserts, soft drinks and beverages. The astringent essential oil, cold-extracted from the fresh peel, is non-toxic, non-irritant, non-sensitising and unharmed by sunlight. It has a short shelf life as it oxidises quickly. It is used as a tonic in skincare, e.g. for acne and congested oily skin, and as a toner for flaccid facial skin and tissues. Often used in cellulite massage, oedema and obesity, the oil is said to be stimulating to the lymphatic system and to digestion. It is also used in pre-exercise products and is useful for post-exercise conditions such as muscle fatigue, performance stress (especially athletic) and stiffness, as well as nervous exhaustion. It is spirit-lifting and alleviates nervous conditions such as headache and depression. Being bactericidal, it is also useful against chills, colds and flu.

CALENDULA / MARIGOLD
Calendula officinalis
S. EUROPE& MEDITERRANEAN

One of the most common colourants used in processed foods we eat the active ingredients of the Pot Marigold or Calendula every day. This pungent herb is an ingredient in many different skin preparations, cosmetics and toiletries; (the leaves were used to make washes for sore eyes). It is employed throughout Europe to treat all kinds of skin problems ranging from bee stings to frostbite. It is commonly used externally as an ointment or cream for cuts, bruises, grazes, wounds, acne, rashes, burns, scalds, red, inflamed skin, sunburn and general minor skin conditions Calendula soap has been shown to be an effective cleansing agent for allergy sufferers. Marigold has a mild oestrogenic action that may be used to help decrease period pain and regulate menstrual bleeding. Its anti-fungal properties are often made use of in an infusion 'douche' for vaginal thrush. However, its ability to cause uterine contractions makes it unsuitable for use in pregnancy

Marigold has long been used to reduce inflammations and fever, to stimulate the immune system and the production of bile. It is thought to retard tumour growth and also to tranquillize the central nervous system. Long considered a detoxifying herb, it actively addresses the underlying toxicity of infections and their ensuing fevers. It is also a diuretic and used to combat water retention.

Scientifically, it is a proven wound healer, however, its active agents remain unclear. The flowers' extracts and oil exhibit definite antimicrobial, antifungal and antiviral effects and definitively heal the skin. Triterpenoids are shown as the most important anti-inflammatory agent in the drug and faradiol monoester appears to be the most relevant among it's properties. Calendula may also prove useful in liver disease and infection or erosion in the upper digestive tracts. The carotenoid content of the plant, (including flavoxathin and auroxanthin), may well account in part for its significant free radical scavenging and antioxidant activity. However, it should not be used by those individuals allergic to the daisy family.

The light of scientific research is revealing the fact that this humble pot plant puts more than a little colour back into our cheeks.

WITCHAZEL.
Hamamelis virginiana
NEW WORLD

Long used in North America as a soothing wash for burns, scrapes and bruises, Witchazel is a great shrub to grow in the garden filling the winter air with its soothing fragrance. The medicinal value of 'Witchazel' was known to many of the first tribal people of America. The Mohawk used the bark as a wash for sore eyes and as a compress for painful swellings through the astringent tightening up of capillaries caused by its content of tannins. Witchazel is especially good for reducing inflammations and is widely used as an external treatment for spots, skin blemishes, sore nipples, bruises and sprains. It is used commercially in eyedrops, lotions, skin tonics, skin creams, aftershaves and in other cosmetic preparations. Witchazel is also used internally for diarrhoea. Recent research and studies show that witchazel contains antioxidants, polyphenol compounds, and polysaccharides. Also proanthrocyanidins which reduce water loss via the skin, erythema formation and aid skin treatments significantly. The extract is highly regarded in treating stomach or lungs haemorrhages, haemorrhoids and varicose veins. It also regulates bleeding, mucous secretions and discharges. (A proven antiseptic useful for inclusion in antimicrobial products.) New research shows that among 28 plants tested regarding their effectiveness in peroxynitrite scavenging activity, Witchhazel's hamamelitannin was found to be the most efficacious suggesting that it might be developed as a preventive against such free radical proliferated coronary diseases.

A NICE HEAD OF HAIR

Hair is one of the main features that distinguish mammals from all other warm-blooded animals. Even whales and dolphins have some, and most land mammals are covered in the stuff. Hair is made of that very special protein called keratin; it consists of two layers, a protective outer one and an inner coloured one. Between the two is a cortex made of amino-acid chains, which give the main bounce to your hair. The outer layer is made up of tiny scales which, when your hair is healthy, lie flat, reflecting the light and giving you that glossy, well groomed look.

Each hair consists of a club-shaped root embedded in a follicle, grows about 25 centimetres a year, and lasts for only three to five years before it falls out. At any one time 75 per cent of your hair is growing and 25 per cent is withering; not surprisingly, it's the latter which tends to fall out. Replacements grow from new follicles formed in your skin. (Hair transplants consist of moving tiny bits of skin with active follicles from a hairy spot into a bald spot.) An average blond has about 150,000 hairs on his or her head, a redhead 90,000 and the rest of us somewhere in between – that is, until we start to go bald. Natural hair care comes thanks to the sebaceous glands, which produce the original grease conditioning the hair and the scalp. Two natural products also appear to be particularly effective: sperm-whale oil, which no civilised person would now think of using, and jojoba (pronounced 'hohoba') liquid wax.

Permanent baldness may well be genetically determined and is, as its name suggests, permanent, and the onset can be as early as the age of fifteen. So the only advice is, if you have it, sit back and enjoy it! Revel in all those bald wrestlers, admire Yul Brynner and don't forget the widely held belief that baldness is a sign of virility.

Also remember that it's easier to change your hat than the colour of your hair. Going grey is not only genetically determined, it is also a sign of growing old. The mature silverback gorilla is king of the pack, the ladies love him. Grey, white, silver – there's a hidden meaning in a name, and whatever you do to hide it the roots will never lie. What's more, chemical dyes and blue rinses, not to mention hot curlers, are unfortunately not counted among the best hair tonics. The hair-care litmus test is that the healthier your hair, the quicker the roots will show their true colours.

Ever since the first stage production of the musical *South Pacific* in which the leading lady had to wash her hair on stage every night except Sundays and twice on matinée days, every hair-care product company has done their best with shampoos and conditioners. Suffice to say that in India and Sri Lanka, both renowned for fantastic heads of hair, daily washing is a ritual, with soap and water. However, each wash does remove some of the skin's outer layers of cells and if the correct balance isn't struck then dandruff, tiny flakes of dead skin, will tell the world there's something wrong.

It has often been said that your hair is the barometer of your state of health. Old wives' tale? Well, take a look in the mirror next time you have a hangover or a cold. Remember your hair is there to protect your head from the elements, so a good dose of honest-to-goodness sunshine and rain cannot do it too much harm. Wearing hats all the time and living in centrally heated homes, air-conditioned offices and aeroplanes, let alone using hair-dryers at full blast, does exactly the opposite. My advice is let it all hang out as often as you can, and use rainwater for washing. A rainwater butt provides a free supply and gives you your own mini-wetland habitat right in your own back yard.

The hair we see when we look in the mirror is technically dead, and we may think that all we can do to improve its looks is to add cosmetics, which often means just plastering them on. But let's get to the root of it all. Hair care, like body care, begins with diet; so if your health barometer shows hot and dry, don't treat the symptoms – treat the cause. Choose your hair-care products with the care your hair deserves, and check back to Chapter 2 (on diet), for barometers never lie.

The rate at which our hair turns grey is due to the reduced activity of an enzyme called tyrosinase that regulates the amount of melanin produced in the hair's pigment cells. Tyrosinase activity is related to prostaglandin production, and may be improved by increasing our intake of essential fatty acids. Most types of hair loss appear to be governed at least in part by the male hormone testosterone, and both males and females can suffer from an imbalance of this hormone. Dandruff is also a hormone-related problem, and attacks are often triggered by stress. So in order to make the hormones flow and the enzymes get to work you need a good diet that includes vitamin E, fish oil, nuts, fresh fruit and vegetables, and onions. Onions are rich in sulphur and that's what holds all those keratin molecules together. Butter and hard margarines are high in saturated fats so should be avoided, and although high-polyunsaturated spreads *are* made with polyunsaturates, their structure is usually changed by hydrogenation. In this process hydrogen is bonded into the oil molecules to change their structure from a liquid into a solid fat. Hydrogenation destroys the health benefits of the oils, so it is worth seeking out unhydrogenated spreads from healthfood shops.

JOJOBA
Simmondsia chinensis
NEW WORLD

Jojoba originated in the deserts of Mexico and has become a cause célèbre in the field of conservation, for it does all the things sperm-whale oil used to be used for and in some cases does them better. And with the cultivation of jojoba across the world there is even less argument for the 'sustainable' harvesting of sperm-whales. Jojoba fruits are a rich source of polyunsaturated oil that not only thickens and so conditions the hair, helping to stop excessive loss, but also prevents over-secretion by the sebaceous glands and hence the excessive build-up of sebum on the scalp.

Jojoba oil needs minimal refining and has specific skincare properties. Soothing and softening, and with a chemical composition close to the skin's own (sebum), at body temperature it 'melts' swiftly when rubbed on to the skin. This natural affinity with human skin makes it usable by all skin types. Research shows that the unsaponifiables contained in all vegetable oils (jojoba's content has 50 per cent), when applied to the skin, increase the effect of the body's own stretchy stuff, elastin. Deterioration of elastin comes with age and overexposure to the sun. Used externally for dry skin and hair, acne, psoriasis and sunburn, jojoba oil is especially good for sensitive complexions, delicate or oily, and has bactericidal properties that resist spoilage and rancidity. Thorough cleansing of the skin before application of the oil preparation is essential, and long-term use is advised. Jojoba is naturally pH-balanced. For a beneficial treatment of dry or bleached hair, and for scalp and hair cleansing, massage the oil into the scalp and hair; leave for fifteen minutes before shampooing and conditioning.

COCONUT
Cocos nucifera
PACIFIC

In Tahiti, coconut oil is used by the Polynesians as a base in which to macerate gardenia flowers (*Gardenia tahitensis*) to make *monoi* (a preparation made mainly of coconut oil and gardenia flowers). It is used in aromatherapeutic massage and for beauty preparations and has very good psychological and skincare effects. Coconut oil has probably been a medicinal and beauty treatment of the people living in and around the tropical islands and coasts for longer than recorded time. Living often in harsh, sunny conditions, South Sea Islanders are envied for their glossy locks and smooth, supple skin. Cosmetically, emollient coconut oil gives a satin-smooth finish to the skin. It also aids tanning, but does not filter the sun's rays. Used in massage and as a body dressing by canoe racers prior to racing, coconut oil reputedly tones the muscles, smoothes the skin and gives energy and added virility. It is interesting that those racers who anoint their hair with coconut oil from childhood seldom go grey or bald.

In India the coconut is considered to be the fruit for a long and healthy life, and in Ayurvedic medicine it is used for treating burns and dissolving kidney-stones, and for heart and circulatory problems and hair loss. The fractionated oil, containing triacyl-glycerols, is used in the diets of patients with cystic fibrosis because it is more easily absorbed by the gastrointestinal tract. It is also used in suppositories because it softens and melts at body temperature. Fractionated oil, which is not the complete oil, is what is mostly sold in the West, as the oil can cause an allergic reaction in some people.

Researchers over nearly four decades have found the lauric acid in coconut to be antiviral and antibacterial, and it has certain antiprotozoal properties useful in the treatment of diseases such as HIV, herpes and listeria. Also, coconut's capric acid has an antiviral effect on herpes simplex, and a bactericidal effect on chlamydia and other sexually transmitted diseases. Recent testing on animals shows that the lipid composition of coconut fats puts them at the top of the league when it comes to helping iron make itself available in the blood. So they are especially recommended for infant formulas. Coconut protein reduces hyperlipidaemia and some of the worse effects of a high-cholesterol diet.

6

Foot-loose and Fancy-free – and Give Them a Big Hand!

ONE PAIR OF FEET

That's all you've got, and they're going to have to last you for life, however heavy you get. One of the main problems with modern-day feet is that we tend to keep them shut away in socks and shoes. This does them little good. So let them out whenever you can, and take a walk on the wild side.

No outdoor trim-track is really complete without a rough grassy area (regularly cleared of dog-dirt, ring-pulls and glass) for foot work-outs. Try it out on the lawn at home and see how it soothes after a long day at work. Going barefoot around the house also makes good sense, and toe-wiggling and foot press-ups while seated, especially on aeroplanes, do wonders for the circulation and the underworked muscles and bones of the feet. Exposure to the air, especially when exercising, allows the feet to sweat and so cleanses the body of many waste substances which, as you know to your cost, can cause an awful stink.

One thing you should never try to do is suppress this natural process using chemicals of any sort. The simple answer is to wash and thoroughly dry your feet as regularly as possible; the drying is very important because all life depends on water, and that includes the fungi and bacteria that cause foot rot. Best of all is the *Chariots of Fire* method, running along the beach and in and out of the sea, then a final spurt above the high-tide mark to let the sand dry them off. You'll be surprised how quickly your feet will toughen up, and you'll soon be able to tackle the pebbles without a hobble or a flinch.

The music-hall figure of the rubicund colonel sitting in a wicker-work wheelchair screaming abuse at the child who has just bumped into his gout-ridden foot may be a thing of the past. But not so the disease, which is once again on the rampage amongst our more self-indulgent citizens. Earl Mindell, one of America's greatest contemporary exponents of herbal healing, gives some frightening statistics in his book *Secret Remedies* published in 1997: 'Over two million Americans suffer the excruciating pain and swelling of gout. More than 95 per cent of gout sufferers are men over the age of thirty. The number of Americans with this disorder has doubled over the past thirty years.'

Gout is a form of arthritis, caused by a defect in the way uric acid is broken down by the body. The result is an excess of uric acid salts accumulating in and around the joints, especially those of the big toe. Too much uric acid can also damage the kidneys and lead to the formation of kidney stones. It is now known that this troublesome acid is a by-product of the breakdown of purine, so food high in this amino acid should be avoided. These include asparagus, bran, cauliflower, legumes, liver, mackerel, red meat, sardines, shrimps, eel, spinach and whole grains. I can hear the cry – What is there left to live on, let alone *for*? Well, how about keeping a food diary and let your big toe be your barometer. You may well find that certain foods are the main triggers.

Today the typical treatment for gout involves the use of prescription drugs that increase the excretion of uric acid, or which slow the formation of uric acid salts. If you have severe gout, these can help relieve your symptoms. And here are some other supplements and foods that may help to prevent another flare-up. Cherries can lower uric-acid levels, and cherry juice is used in Europe as a bona fide treatment for gout. Other helpful fruits include blueberries, juniper berries, and other dark-red or -blue berries – in fact, all those 'fruits of the forest', to use a supermarket term. These berries are rich in a whole portfolio of antioxidants believed to help normalise uric-acid levels. In nature they are available just at the right time, as the more sedentary life of winter approaches and as many people turn to alcohol for winter warmth and comfort.

As I type, the papers are overflowing with tales of DVT (deep-vein thrombosis) woe. Just as the long northern winter may trigger a bad dose of the DTs, as our grandmothers would have said, it would appear that our ever more sedentary year-round lifestyles may be the cause of deep-vein thrombosis. One trigger is said to be long-haul flights spent cooped up in economy-class seats, with major hospitals close to Heathrow getting at least two long-haul cases per week. East Surrey Health Authority, whose hospitals cover Gatwick, recorded 142 DVT deaths between April 1999 and April 2000. But compare this to the fact that DVT in Britain claims the lives of thirty thousand people a year, many of whom die as a result of high-risk factors such as heart disease, smoking and immobility.

High fliers, the Saga set, desk jockeys and even telly and PlayStation addicts, beware: don't just wait to ignore the government health warnings on economy-class tickets – take your lifestyles more seriously. When travelling by car, bus, train or cruise liner, or flying any class, remember, take en route exercise and make sure you drink plenty of mineral water. Those who find they suffer from incontinence as a result of taking my advice could ask the airlines concerned to increase the number of toilets, but that would cut down the exercise time spent standing in the queue. The solution to lifestyle syndromes is never simple.

CHERRY
Prunus avium and other spp.
EUROPE

The cherry provides dietary fibre and is virtually fat- and cholesterol-free. It contains no starch, and is low in sugar and protein, but is jam-packed with vitamins. Potassium-rich, it lowers uric acid levels and makes an excellent food medicine as well as a juicy remedy for arthritic conditions such as gout. Today many gout sufferers testify that cherry juice and eating cherries give them as much relief as commonly prescribed anti-gout drugs. Both wild and domesticated cherries contain cyanogenic glycosides in their leaves, bark and stones – all of interest to pharmacologists. Michigan State University's research indicates that the anti-inflammatory properties of tart cherry compounds are at least ten times more active than aspirin, but without any of the adverse side-effects. Indeed, eating only twenty cherries a day could reduce inflammatory pain and headache.

Highly antioxidant, red and black cherries provide antho-cyanins, known to be anti-carcinogenic. Ripe sweet cherries (*P. avium*) also contain a flavonoid (beta-glucosidase), a compound that may reduce the likelihood of developing degenerative dis-eases. Tart cherries contain more melatonin, an antioxidant that helps destroy free radicals and is usually produced in the brain's pineal gland (which controls sleeping and waking), than is nor-mally found in the blood. Research at the University of Iowa has shown that tart cherries also contain perillyl alcohol (POH), a natural compound that is powerful in reducing the incidence of all types of cancer by depriving them of essential proteins, so shutting down their growth. In animal tests, POH has been shown to be five times more potent than other known cancer-reducing compounds at inducing tumour regression in advanced carcinomas of the breast, prostate and ovary.

No side-effects have been reported from concentrated cherry juice, although allergic reactions are always possible and overindulgence even in a good thing can produce stomach ache. All in all, cherry juice is a fine example of folkloric herbalism and modern medicine coming together, but there is still a long way to go.

GIVE THEM A BIG HAND

Next time you are applauding your favourite soloist playing his or her instrument to perfection, spare a thought for all the neuro-hardware invested in that stunning display of dexterity, for our hands are equipped with an enormous number of nerve cells. Add to this the large amount of brain set aside to deal with and process all that digi-tised information, and it is little wonder that Pac-Man started the PlayStation revolution.

All nerve cells are made of omega-3 and omega-6 unsaturated fatty acids in a fifty-fifty mixture, and our fingers require a regular supply of these throughout our lifetime. It's hardly surprising, then, that when we clog the system with too much cholesterol our fingers react with arthritis. Indeed, if it gets very bad or if we suffer — and that's the appropriate word – from peripheral vascular disease, our fingers curl and our hands become club-like, almost like hoofs.

Animals with hoofs don't have the same problem, and all have very small brains relative to their size. Horses, for example, have brains that take up only 0.05 per cent of their total body weight, compared to 2 per cent in us humans. Horses are total herbivores, eating vast amounts of leafy plant material, which is a very poor source of those brain- and nerve-building unsaturates. It is, of course, full of indigestible roughage, so they do produce high-class manure. Cows have more complex feet and larger brains than horses. It may come as a shock but they are not strict herbivores let alone vegans. Like all ruminants they chew the cud, and have a complex digestive system in which bacteria and protozoa live and help to digest even the roughest roughage. That's why cowpats are only second-class fertiliser and why cows, sheep and goats should be called omnivores. The fact is they digest billions of tiny animals with every burp, producing the explosive greenhouse gas methane at the same time.

Then why, you might ask, don't cows have really big brains? The fact is that in the depths of the cow's stomach, which acts as a fermentation vat, there is no oxygen. In consequence, all the waste hydrogen produced during the digestive process gets tacked on to the fats, saturating them. Poor old cow – insufficient unsaturates to build a big brain and plenty of cholesterol to dump in store in those T-bones and other juicy steaks.

Perhaps strangest of all in this fat tale of woe is that much of the problem is of recent occurrence and of our own making. The meat of wild animals does not overflow with saturated fat; in fact, they are a great source of polyunsaturates. All our domestic stock started their lives this way; always on the move, running and roaming across the plains, they stored very little in the way of fat except in readiness for winter. However, in recent years we have more and more shut them up in fields and byres away from their original varied diet of leafy twigs, seeds and fruits and fed them on concentrated energy – even, in the case of cows, on their own offal. We have made them cannibals, so no wonder some went mad. The sad truth is that we have now done the same to all our main livestock, even to our pigs and battery hens, all of which should now be labelled with a government health warning.

Although this is a book about herbal medicine the following

species of free-range animals deserve a mention, given the world war now being waged against too much bad cholesterol. These animals (and birds) all provide meat that is low in saturated fats and yet has more than its fair share of the polyunsaturated goodies. What is more, the first four, where properly managed, do help maintain biodiverse rural landscapes, and are key players in the economy that supports them and used to support us.

Managing even the best organic farm requires the destruction of the habitat of many wild animals and the continued culling of those that would eat the crops. It can be done using either poison or guns. So in my view, the ethical management of our countryside must include well trained gamekeepers. (Then we can forget about poison.) I have long been a campaigner against the inhumanities of veal crates and of the battery-farming of chickens, turkeys and ducks. But please, those of you who are vegetarians, before you start to get hot under the collar, consider the number of animals and birds that must be culled to ensure that your plates are full. And then let's be clear that the organic method, though infinitely preferable, has its down side, too.

PHEASANT
Phasianus colchicus
ASIA

A well managed estate producing these handsome game-birds is a patchwork of mature and coppiced woodland, small fields complete with hedgerows; pastures, meadows and arable fields. All in all an ideal habitat, not only for the pheasants but also for a whole cross-section of our native wildlife and wild flowers. Most of these have in recent years been swept away, replaced by enormous fields of cereals, home of the combine, spray boom and farm subsidies. Free-range pheasants are a tribute to rural Britain – like battery hens the recent development of 'battery pheasants' estates mismanaged for short term profits with no respect of to animal welfare are an abomination and must be banned.

GREY PARTRIDGE
Perdix perdix
ENGLAND

The work of the Game Conservancy at Fordingbridge in the heart of Hardy country, still far from the madding crowd, is showing the way ahead. This includes a place for free-range partridges as a key part of broader-based farming employing fewer chemicals and with more woods and marginal land overflowing with butterflies, other insects, wild flowers and jubilations (this is the correct word!) of skylarks singing the praises of good economic sense.

RED GROUSE
Lagopus scoticus
GREAT BRITAIN

This is Britain's only endemic bird, which means (in the stricter sense) that it is found nowhere else in the world. Its habitat, the moorlands footing our mountains, has long been under threat from the massive planting of conifers in the wrong place and the overgrazing of sheep (which are dipped in highly toxic chemicals before being transported many stressful miles to a slaughterhouse). Today in many areas the only thing that keeps our uplands clad in heather, which gives us the added benefit of arguably the best honey in the world, is the work of the gamekeepers. And more about that honey: recent reports show that organic honey contains substances that can kill superbugs. Great news indeed, especially since it's also reported that one year down the line deadly superbugs have already developed resistance to the much lauded synthetic antibiotic linezolid.

Because of our modern way of agricultural life, the next two species have taken on the role of vermin whose populations must be strictly controlled, at least as a damage-limiting operation – again, this must be the work of well trained gamekeepers.

RABBIT
Oryctolagus cuniculus
EUROPE

In the days before *Watership Down* and myxomatosis, trainloads of wild rabbits ready for the table used to arrive in London every day through spring to autumn. The trains often carried other game-birds and venison – as much as 60,000 tonnes a year – for that more gourmet market. This extra harvest helped the farmers in their constant battle to keep in business, both economically and ecologically.

RED DEER
Cervus elaphus
EUROPE

There are now an estimated 250,000 too many hinds in Scotland, and the 'monarch of the glen' has taken on a new and devastating role in the local ecology and economy – as destroyer of the little that is left of the once great forest of Caledon and of the livelihood of many crofters. Expert culling programmes are absolutely necessary, and the lean free-range organic meat makes a lot of sense to those of us addicted to omnivory, but who still hanker after a more healthful diet.

The same is true, sadly, of all the world's game and game-birds. As Eve's growing family moved out across the world they destroyed the megafauna wherever they went. The miracle of that story is that of all the continents and islands they colonised, only Africa retained viable populations of most of its big game. But the current exploding population of Africa is changing all that. Squeezed into ever-smaller areas, many species of game both big and small are now in danger of extinction. The reason is all too often the replacement of traditional ways of life, which included hunting (the original form of culling) the local game for their lean meat, with cash crops and fatstock.

7

Healthy in Heart

It was the invention of cheap and reliable pumps that made modern small-bore central-heating systems possible. Likewise, it was the evolution of a four-chambered heart (in which blood returning from the body depleted of oxygen, and oxygen-rich blood recharged by the lungs, could be kept completely separate) which allowed the real success of the warm-blooded mammals. The crocodile clan had pioneered the design and some dinosaurs may well have had something almost as efficient, but it was the endotherms, the warm-blooded ones, that perfected this particular hunk of muscle. Your heart muscle, or myocardium, is hard at work from your first heartbeat eight months before you are born until the day you die.

Ba-dum, ba-dum, the double-beat rhythm of life. It's this pulse that keeps the blood pressure high enough to supply all the parts of your body with all the oxygen, nutrients and energy it needs, while moving wastes out to the liver, kidneys and skin where they can be dealt with. Made of very special cardiac muscle, the sort that never gets tired and yet can contract rapidly, your heart is about the size of a loosely clenched fist. Weighing in at about 300 grams, with a power requirement of 0.003 horsepower, it is the thing that above all else allows champions to become champions. At rest our hearts beat around seventy times a minute – that's an incredible 2.9 billion beats in eighty years, which is now the average life expectancy of someone living in the rich First World. Fantastic, especially when research indicates that most other mammals die once their hearts have beaten 1.5 billion times.

The lifespan of our hunting-gathering ancestors was about forty years – much nearer the 1.5 billion heartbeat mark than their modern counterparts. It would be nice to think that we are becoming super-mammals, but the more probable explanation of our postmodern swinging success is that unlike wild animals we don't have to rush about all the time searching for and catching food, or running away to avoid things that want to eat us. So we have energy to spare to keep our hearts and blood systems in good repair. The problem is, all this sitting about can make us fat, putting extra strain on our hearts. So it's little wonder that poor diets increase the likelihood of heart disease.

Heart attack is one of the most dreaded facts of modern life, because it is the thing that kills most of us off. Myocardial infarction, for that is the official name of the commonest form, is in all probability going to be the epitaph on our death certificate. Myocardial infarction. Sounds awful, doesn't it? – like some last rectal whimper. And it's no good saying, 'I don't want to go like that', because you have got to go somehow. However good a dietary life you may think you have led, even a non-smoking, non-drinking vegan has got to die sometime. When the time comes, a hiccup in your myocardium is probably the best way out. Myocardial infarction should be looked upon as a fitting, final fanfare for the common man or woman when their heart has run its allotted lifespan.

GOOD DIETS, NOT-SO-GOOD DIETS, AND CHOLESTEROL

We are often told that among people living in primitive societies heart attack is not the main cause of death. But the fact is that in many cases they don't live as long as we do, so they can't suffer our 'diseases' of old age. They also die of some pretty nasty things that our lifestyles allow us to avoid. However, there is much evidence that as they take on our ways of living, they also get hooked with our ways of dying. Studies of the populations of a number of developed countries are throwing light on the matter. Heart attack is not a common cause of premature death in countries like Japan and Italy, but as they are being weaned onto a more, for want of a better term, 'milk-and-red-fat diet' things appear to be shifting in the wrong direction – fast.

The Japanese diet traditionally includes lots of fish and shellfish, beans, peas and other pulses, grains and soya-based products like tofu. Their staple was brown rice, and they ate little in the way of red meat or dairy products until 1931 when the first herd of cows was introduced. They were not great wine or beer drinkers, but did sip a little sake. In fact, everything in the Japanese dietary garden was OK until Western influences began to infiltrate their market-place.

On the other hand the traditional Italian diet, which staples on pasta, sweet chestnut and garlic, swims in olive oil and red wine. It also comes with lots of red meat: salami, prosciutto and bresaola for starters; then pasta with cheese, veal or steak for the main course, and great fresh salads. Followed by black coffee – never cappuccino. When it comes to stress, they let it out vociferously and then become their laid-back selves again.

Another feature of the Mediterranean diet is that wedge of lemon as a garnish for both fish and meat. Also, real lemonades like the Spanish *grenissada de limón* are thought to help thin the blood. Then there are those pine kernels, an integral part of many dishes. They are traditionally eaten as gather-your-own snacks by children running wild, as all children used to do in the fields and woodlands. Pine kernels contain large amounts of vitamin E, all great for the young in heart, as well as B_1 and high levels of iron and other minerals to store against old age. Likewise, the anticoagulant resin that exudes from pine trunks is used in a variety of traditional sweets: try the French *suc des Vosges* and do yourself no harm at all, for the resin contains pycnogenol, an analgesic. According to Professor Ronald Watson of the University of Arizona School of Medicine in *Cardiology Review and Reports* (June 1999), pycnogenol is 'a safe and natural option, especially for those who cannot tolerate the adverse effects of aspirin'.

So what *is* wrong with our diets? What really raises the likelihood of a heart attack? Well, it all appears to revolve around those dreaded saturated fatty acids and – dare I mention the word again? – cholesterol. The tabloids overflow with it and so does our fast-food diet, including the fish and chips we used to be allowed to eat out of newspaper. It's to do with highly bred red meat, battery chickens, milk, cream, butter, and all the other products the dairy industry makes from what it skims off skimmed milk.

Beginning to wonder why your body ever bothered with fat at all? But as you'll remember, the answer to that is simple: fats when saturated are the best stores of energy for a shapely body. Take Mr Average, weighing in at 70 kilograms, with 100,000 kilocalories of energy stored as fat, 25,000kcal as protein, mostly in muscle, 600kcal as glycogen and 40kcal as glucose. If that amount of energy were stored as carbohydrate he would have to carry an extra 55kg, whereas saturated fat would make up only 11kg of his total body weight. The original big sugar daddy.

But the fact is that fat, in the form of cholesterol, is an absolutely necessary part of our chemical make-up and without it we would die. Yes, the now dreaded cholesterol plays a key role in the function of the membranes that surround and divide the contents of every cell in our bodies. It is also a major step along the road by which our bodies make steroid hormones, including our sex hormones. In order to keep up a balanced supply to all those cells cholesterol makes up 79 per cent of the low-density lipids carried around in our blood, while high-density lipids take it to the liver for breakdown and excretion. Cholesterol is so important that if we don't get enough in our diets, the liver and the intestines have the ability to make about 800 milligrams of it a day. We can't function without it, but if there's too much in our diets our bodies stop making it, in what we might call a desperate attempt to keep that healthy balance. The problem is that the only way our bodies seem to be able to make us stop taking in too much of it, is to produce a heart attack.

There is now ample proof that people between the ages of thirty-three and forty-four whose blood serum contains more than 256 milligrams per decilitre of cholesterol are five times more likely to be hit by a heart attack than those whose serum levels are less than 220 milligrams per decilitre. New research results are being published all the time, but the message remains the same: not too little, not too much.

The main cause of heart attacks and the cause of ischaemic heart disease – characterised by a slowing-down of the blood flow – is arteriosclerosis, a degenerative condition of the arteries brought about by the build-up of lipids, mainly cholesterol, combined with proteins and bits that have fallen off the artery wall. All this coagulates into porridge-like lumps called 'plaques'. The porridge is stirred, not on the plate but by the blood's platelets, present in abundance in every millilitre of the staff. The platelets' real job in life is to help keep the walls of the blood vessels in good repair. But spurred on by those wicked saturated fats, they help stick the wrong things together, thus contributing to plaque formation.

As the build-up of plaques gradually begins to slow the flow of blood, up goes your blood pressure. Despite the heart doing all it can to compensate, finally the vein or artery becomes blocked. If it's an artery, and if the artery in question supplies blood to the heart, it's a coronary; if to the brain, it's a stroke. In both cases sudden death can result; or, with care, recovery can be the way ahead, but often with some permanent damage.

Any damage to the heart, through accident, contact sports, over-exertion or illness, can leave weak spots, building up trouble for the future. It has been estimated that in the USA the cost of healthcare related to arteriosclerosis is around 56 billion dollars a year – that is, over 1.5 per cent of their GNP. Little wonder that a lot of money is being poured into research. This research shows that it's not only diet but also tobacco and coffee consumption that can crank up the problem. More than six cups of coffee a day can increase serum cholesterol. Black tea doesn't have the same effect, but be careful with the unskimmed milk. Smoking cigarettes brings about a mean increase of 70 per cent in the risk of heart attack and a three- to fivefold increase in the risk of ischaemic heart disease.

Human milk merits the top design award for building human babies, especially their nerve cells and blood vessels, while cow's milk is good for building big bodies, strong bones and lean muscles. Well, it was until someone came up with what, in hindsight, was a not so bright idea: namely, that as weight was the thing that really mattered in the marketplace, feeding cows with offal spiced up with treated human sewage was the thing to do; and it would also solve the problem of waste disposal while increasing profits. When it comes to humans, it's the nomadic Masai people of Kenya and Tanzania who enjoy and thrive on what should be regarded as the world's most unhealthy diet. John Beutler, a chemist from the National Cancer Research Institute, Bethesda, USA, is fascinated by the fact that 'the Masai have a diet that has nothing in it that is good for you, such as fruit, fish or fibre. They eat meat, blood and cow's milk, all bad things.' They consume up to 2,000 milligrams of cholesterol a day and yet maintain a healthy blood cholesterol level, about one-third that of an average affluent male American. Genetics cannot be the whole answer, for as they are forced to change their nomadic lifestyles and live in towns, up go their cholesterol levels. Although the nomadic life makes for lean animals and lean meat, sadly the same is not true of the stock of ordinary beef farmers. Research is now being directed at a number of the Masai's own brand of food additives – the bark of certain trees, especially *Albizia anthelmintica* and *Acacia goetzii* – which may contain substances with cholesterol-lowering properties. One day these barks may help us to bite on meat without misgivings, if not with vegan ethics.

Already more than one hundred plants, including many members of the pea flower family, are known to contain saponins which are thought to bind cholesterol, keeping it within the gut so that it just passes on through. But until some of these, or the Kalahari Bushmen's hunger-stopper the Hoodia cactus (see p. 85), come on to the market, here are a few tips straight from the American Food and Nutrition Board's mouth:

To avoid heart disease and stroke:
(1) Stop smoking.
(2) Exercise – walk for twenty minutes five times per week.
(3) Eat less meat and fried foods.
(4) Eat more fruits and vegetables and fibrous foods.
(5) Have a regular cholesterol check.
(6) Keep body weight under control (extra body fat increases risk of heart disease).

OLIVE
Olea europaea
MEDITERRANEAN

Originating in, and today the hallmark of, the Mediterranean region, the oil expressed from ripe olive fruits has been used in cooking, medicine and even surgery for more than six thousand years. Rich in unsaturated fatty acids and with almost no cholesterol, low in saturates and with a calorific value higher than butter – *and* full of vitamin A, folic acid, calcium and phosphate – olive oil may hold one of the keys to Italy's enviably low standing in the coronary stakes. In conjunction with highly antioxidant red wine, garlic, onions and tomatoes, olive oils are well known to be instrumental in balancing the 'bad' LDL cholesterol with the 'good' HDL cholesterol levels in the body, thereby alleviating heart conditions. Scientific studies conclude that a large amount of olive oil in the diet is anticoagulant and so protects against heart attack. If you don't believe that quality counts, you'll be interested to hear that research reveals that extra virgin olive oil (the first cold-pressing) contains phenolic compounds such as hydroxytyrosol and oleuropein, which are not only responsible for its pungent taste and high stability but are powerful antioxidants too.

Long a symbol of peace, security and plenty, the olive leaf was probably first used by the ancients in the mummification of their pharaohs. Later, in other cultures, olive leaf extracts were employed as a common folklore remedy to relieve fevers. In recent times, Italian researchers have found that oleuropein, also found in the leaf, has the capacity to lower blood pressure in animals. Other European researchers have confirmed this, also finding that olive leaf extract increases blood flow in the coronary arteries and relieves irregular heartbeat. From the evidence of clinical trials, olive leaf appears to be able to lower the LDL level by 30 per cent or more, without exercise or extreme dietary changes. The more olive leaf extract is investigated, the more its attributes accumulate: it is a new and revolutionary treatment for heart disease, diabetes, arthritis, herpes (*Herpes zoster*) and chronic fatigue. Recent research is looking into the use of olive leaf's antioxidant power to increase the shelf life of food products instead of using synthetics, while investigating its possible protective effect in human cells. It could, perhaps, be said that olive leaf extract has a very heartening future.

Self-medication should not be undertaken for any serious diseases. Some individuals may experience adverse reactions to the use of olive leaf.

GARLIC
Allium sativum

CENTRAL ASIA

The spice of life is garlic. The storage organs of this member of the lily family, unlike all the other onions, develop entirely under ground, and have been cultivated for at least four thousand years. We know that during the construction of the pyramids the slaves were fed with enormous amounts of garlic. The Egyptian medical papyri tell us of the use of this pungent cure for all manner of complaints, from insect bites to wounds (one presumes they also included their own form of whiplash injury).

Modern research has shown that garlic can lower blood cholesterol, that it improves the general health of the heart and blood system, and may help stabilise blood sugar levels. There are some 2,200 scientific research papers and publications proving that garlic supports the cardiovascular system. While eating ten or more raw cloves per day can be toxic and in some cases can trigger an allergic reaction, garlic is highly antioxidant, scavenging for the free radicals that attack and destroy bodily tissues at the cellular level. The combined attributes of garlic suggest that it may prevent atherosclerosis, as indicated by the fact that the consumption of 900 milligrams of active garlic supplement has been shown to reduce arterial plaque formation by 5–18 per cent. Garlic has also been shown to have a protective effect on the elastic properties of the aorta in the elderly, and to reduce the symptoms of cramping in the lower legs secondary to poor blood flow. The latter is particularly topical, given recent fears over the link between long-haul flights and deep-vein thrombosis. So garlic each day could help to keep those thromboses at bay, perhaps also proving that your partner is after you and not your money.

Garlic is a useful anti-cancer agent, protecting against stomach, bladder and colorectal cancers and tumour proliferation. Although the compound ajoene has proven useful against acute myeloid leukaemia 'in vitro' – in the laboratory – recent research into garlic's other natural compounds indicates that diallyl disulfide may be the pivotal molecule on which its chemopreventative action against cancer is based. Garlic's stimulation of the immune system and other beneficial effects reduce the incidence of cancer. It has also been shown to be effective against even some antibiotic-resistant strains of the stomach ulcerative *Helicobacter pylori* and other bacterial infections. Furthermore, the first scientific trial of a compound containing pure dried allicin has shown that people taking this garlic extract supplement are less likely to catch a common cold and recover faster if infected.

The latest research advises that garlic may not be taken with anticoagulants, anti-platelet agents or drugs prescribed for hypoglycaemic conditions. Garlic supplements may also impede HIV medication. Life becomes even more complicated as more interactions between new drugs and herbal extracts and concentrates are being discovered. If in doubt seek professional advice.

HAWTHORN
Crataegus monogyna

EUROPE

Don't hedge your bets – all those old wives' tales like 'Ne'er cast a clout 'til May is out' may well have some substance. Long used as a heart tonic, hawthorn has been shown to improve cardiac health and stabilise blood pressure by dilating the blood vessels and increasing cardiac action. Since the Middle Ages, it has been used in Europe as a heart remedy and a traditional medicine, but it has only recently been taken up by the scientific world for investigation and validation.

The main clinical applications of hawthorn are in the long-term treatment of loss of cardiac function – in fact any condition characterised by a feeling of congestion and oppression in the heart area, and mild arrhythmias. Because it is relatively non-toxic, does not accumulate in the body or habituate the individual, it is especially useful for conditions of the ageing heart that do not warrant the use of digitalis (foxglove-based) drugs, such as angina pectoris and coronary artery disease. The hawthorn leaf is also used as a preventive measure against the stable condition of angina, which is caused by a shortage of oxygen in the heart muscle. However, it is slow-acting, so is not a remedy for an acute attack.

Research has found hawthorn to be capable of expanding blood vessels and enabling more oxygen-rich blood to reach the muscles of the heart, thereby boosting heartbeat. This vasodilatory action also aids the heart by reducing resistance elsewhere in the circulatory system. Some of the plant's remedial actions are thought to be due to the amines present.

Congestive heart failure is a serious condition and requires expert management, so don't undertake self-medication. Some individuals – in particular, those hypersensitive to other members of the rose flower family – may experience adverse reactions to hawthorn, such as fatigue, nausea and sweating. High doses of the herb may interact with prescribed anti-hypertensive drugs if taken in conjunction, causing hypotension and intensifying the effect of digoxin, the poison present in the foxglove.

GRAPE
Vitis Vinifera
MEDITERRANEAN, EUROPE

Wine is probably the second-oldest alcoholic drink in human history, and grapes are prized everywhere (as honey must have been the first sweetener, mead may claim pole position in the hangover stakes.) Nicholas Culpeper endorsed the use of the grapevine extract as a mouthwash and stated that ash from burning the the vines helps to whiten the teeth. In traditional European herbal medicine the grapevine has been tapped for remedies against excessive menstruation, menopausal syndrome, haemorrhage, urinary complaints, obesity, cellulite and varicose veins. An age-old Ayurvedic remedy known as *darakchasava*, mainly containing *V. vinifera*, is still prescribed as a cardiotonic. Today, red wine provides plenty of vitamins, minerals and antioxidants – all part of the much lauded healthful Mediterranean diet.

Some thirty long-term studies all agree that moderate alcohol consumption reduces heart attack risk by 25–40 per cent. In the case of red wine, this is due to factors such as the red-pigmented anthocyanins, which help the capillaries. Polyphenols give wine its antioxidants and are also responsible for decreasing the incidence of heart disease among moderate wine drinkers. These phenolic compounds give wine its sharpness and astringency and are the foundation of red wine's long ageing. Some compounds in wine may also inhibit platelet aggregation, which plays a role in the development of coronary heart disease and the hardening of the arteries. Recent research has found anticarcinogenic carotenoids such as beta-carotene and xanthophylls in the musts, berries, skin and pulp of port wines. Beta-carotene and lutein are the most abundant carotenoids, being present in the musts of red grape varieties; appreciable amounts of carotenoids are found in young ports.

Drink–driving is certainly a scourge of the motor-car age, and, as mentioned elsewhere in this book, problems of drinking and flying have recently come to the fore in the form of deep-vein thrombosis. Orally administered extract of red vine leaf, now in trial in Germany, has been found to be a safe and effective treatment for mild chronic venous insufficiency (CVI), significantly reducing oedema in the lower legs while alleviating key CVI-related symptoms. The oedema reduction is at least equivalent to that reported for compression stockings and other oedema-reducing agents. And once you are safely on holiday in the sun, grapes are on hand to help, for the pigments in grapes' dark skin have a photoprotective effect, helping to reduce the amount of cellular damage done by UV radiation. The bitter grapeseed extract ActiVin contains pycnogenols, which act as powerful antioxidants, improving heart function and possibly lowering the chance of heart attack, while decreasing damage to the cardio-vascular system caused by oxidation. So grapes may well be the original package-holiday health deal, and grape-popping a health-ful pastime. It was Leonardo da Vinci who said, 'Grapes are water held together by sunshine.'

Recent research has also shown that more than one daily glass of wine can exacerbate susceptibility to asthma and other allergies; also, that rare individuals may experience exercise-induced anaphylaxis in response to the grape.

ONION
Allium cepa

EUROPE, ASIA

The onion, although a biennial, is grown as an annual for its bulb. A powerhouse of sugar and useful chemicals, it has been used medicinally for millennia. Selected and bred over the years, all types of onions are good for the blood and some are used the world over for respiratory infections such as the common cold, coughs and flu. The characteristic smell of all alliums is caused by sulphur compounds, which have beneficial effects on the cardio-vascular and circulatory systems, as well as on the digestive and respiratory systems.

The common-or-garden onion continues to be a subject of scientific interest and research, as not all its properties or their working mechanisms are known. As a food medicine, raw or cooked onions help protect against the harmful effects of fatty foods. Eating raw onions may help to lower blood cholesterol, and by increasing the levels of HDLs (high-density lipoproteins) help to carry cholesterol away from body tissues and artery walls. Onion also seems to be an anticoagulant, preventing blood clots, as well as increasing the rate at which blood clots are dispersed. It has now been scientifically proved that raw onions are more potent than cooked ones at stopping blood platelets from aggre-gating. Onions have also been found to reduce high blood pres-sure, and to go some way towards offsetting tendencies to angi-na, arteriosclerosis and heart attack. They help to prevent circu-latory diseases such as thrombosis and conditions associated with strokes, thereby reducing the risk of coronary disease. Science has recently assured us that onion is also an antioxidant, the effi-cacy of which is not significantly affected by boiling.

Along with its cousin garlic, onion has also been tested in Egypt for its effect on the egg production of the water-snail that is the intermediate host of the dreaded bilharzia (*Schistosoma mansoni*), a parasite causing one of the most serious of African diseases. The tropical world awaits the results with baited breath.

KUDZU VINE
Pueraria lobata
ASIA, CHINA, JAPAN

Kudzu, also known as 'Japanese arrowroot', is a peculiar plant native to the thickets and forests of China. It has an immense root sometimes reaching the size of the human body, and so is planted in the east to prevent soil erosion and as a fodder crop. In Chinese medicine, kudzu was mentioned in Shen Nong's *Great Herbal* of the first century AD, and used from the sixth century onwards as a remedy for conditions such as muscular pain and measles, and as a safe, effective treatment for alcohol abuse. The latter use is now backed up by research in the USA. Culinarily, the ground root is used in macrobiotic cuisine to thicken sauces. Today, kudzu is known to contain ingredients that lower blood pressure and improve circulation in the muscles of the heart. Chinese research indicates that it increases cerebral blood flow in cases of arteriosclerosis. Closely related species have been investigated for their contraceptive effect.

The active agents diadzin and daidzein (glycosides), which are present in both the roots (*ge gen*) and the flowers (*ge hua*), are responsible for kudzu's effect on the heart and circulatory system. In an animal study both of these substances inhibited the desire for alcohol – good news indeed, for existing drugs that interfere with the way alcohol is metabolised can cause a build-up of toxins. Further investigations into kudzu's anti-alcohol action in humans have yet to be conducted.

RAUWOLFIA
Rauvolfia serpentina

Over two millennia before chlorpromazine was synthesised, ancient India was already using a herbal antipsychotic: *Rauvolfia serpentina*, commonly called 'Indian snakeroot' or *sarpaghandi*, the 'insanity herb' as recorded in the ancient texts of Hindu Ayurvedic medicine. It earned its nickname of 'snakeroot' via its use as an antidote to the bites of poisonous reptiles, and was Mahatma Gandhi's favourite nightcap. Used for centuries in the Caribbean as a sedative, rauwolfia has been shown to contain reserpine, a very useful substance used to combat hypertension. The Swiss company Ciba Geigy brought it on to the market and soon learned to synthesise it, but then found that the natural extract caused fewer patient problems and was cheaper to produce.

In 1931 a paper was published describing the tranquillising and antihypertensive effects of *Rauvolfia serpentina* roots. Because of the drug's noted sedative effects, it was used to treat over a million Indians in the 1940s for high blood pressure. Over the last decade there has been renewed interest in rauwolfia's reserpine component, and low doses of the herb have been found to be effective in treating hypertension. In recent years Russian scientists have also been interested in rauwolfia as a means of combating arrhythmia. Their research focuses on extracting the plant's biologically active compounds, the enzyme superoxide dismutase and an anti-arrhythmic alkaloid called ajmaline.

Do not self-medicate. The whole crude drug is reported to contain some principles that bring about undesirable side-effects such as purgation and sexual debility. Rauwolifia can also make some people drowsy. Nor should it be taken in conjunction with antidepressants such as phenelzine (an MAOI), as it affects these drugs' performances and toxicity.

WALNUT
Juglans regia

EUROPE, ASIA

The humble walnut is packed with nutrients known to lower cholesterol and to reduce the furring-up of the arteries. Researchers in Barcelona have confirmed that eating a Mediterranean diet lowers the risk of heart disease, and if this is combined with eating nine walnuts a day, the risk can be reduced by a further 11 per cent. All nuts are thought to help combat heart disease because they are rich in vitamin E, high-quality protein and essential amino acids, as well as flavonoids and selenium, which are powerful antioxidants. Recent laboratory research demonstrates that walnut polyphenols inhibit the oxidation of plasma and LDLs, and should be considered for use in the treatment of arthritis. Walnuts were chosen for this study because they contain the essential fatty acid omega-3, which we need to maintain healthy cells and transport fats around the body. Unripe walnuts also contain 1300–3000 milligrams of vitamin C per 100 grams – it is these that are used for pickling.

Recent research in Greece has led to the proposal that liposomes isolated from walnut oil may have future applications for the encapsulation and delivery of drugs and the active ingredients of cosmetics. Hitherto, some body-builders have injected the whole fixed oil intramuscularly – a commonly accepted practice – but to ill effect. Studies in Denmark have indicated that such use can lead to tumours and may result in pulmonary complications. So body-builders beware – don't do it.

MAITAKE, JAPANESE MUSHROOM
Grifola frondosa

JAPAN

REISHI, CHINESE MUSHROOM
Ganoderma lucidum

CHINA

The maitake grows deep in the mountains of north-eastern Japan, and is famous for its taste and health benefits. It is also called the 'dancing mushroom' and is produced commercially in Japan and in the United States. Historically, maitake has been used as a tonic and to help the body adapt to stress and support its normal functions. The consumption of the mushroom was thought to prevent high blood pressure, which has been the focal point of modern research. Maitake is also being studied as a potential tool in the management of high cholesterol and obesity. In addition, it is thought to be able to modulate the immune system, and the polysaccharides it contains are under study for their potential role in cancer and AIDS treatment. Research evidence is accruing that maitake extract may be of use in combating 'Type 2' diabetes, which is now becoming the scourge not only of the middle-aged and the elderly but also of obese children.

Reishi mushrooms grow wild on decaying logs and trees in China. They come in several colours, but the red variety is most commonly used and commercially cultivated in northern Japan and Korea. It is used to treat high blood pressure amongst other conditions. Reishi also contains sterols, coumarins and ganoderic acids, which have been shown to decrease low-density lipoprotein (LDL) and triglyceride levels. Ganoderic acids act on blood platelets, reducing the likelihood of their sticking together – an important factor in lowering the risk of heart disease.

Among reishi's many virtues now under the microscope have been found biologically active compounds with potential for protecting cellular DNA from oxidation, and dietary use of reishi may help to prevent colon cancer. Indeed, all the evidence indicates that adding these tasty fungi to your diet may do you a lot of good.

As it may delay the process, reishi is not recommended for those taking blood-thinning medications; pregnant or lactating women should consult a physician.

RED YEAST
Monascus purpureus

Red-yeast extract (RYE) is made by fermenting rice using a red yeast (*Monascus purpureus*). For centuries, the Chinese have used red-yeast rice preparations as a heart remedy. RYE has been studied extensively for the US market; in one particularly important study, the prestigious University College of Los Angeles found that red-yeast extract contains a number of cholesterol-lowering compounds known as statins, among them lovastatin – exactly the same active ingredient that is present in a portfolio of mainstream cholesterol medications. RYE is known to inhibit the action of HMG-CoA reductase, the enzyme the liver employs to make cholesterol, which accounts for approximately 80 per cent of the cholesterol in the body (the rest we obtain from our food).

Because red-yeast extract contains lovastatin the Federal Drugs Administration of the USA tried to ban the brand used in the UCLA study, arguing that it is really a drug, not a herbal remedy. This is a ploy, which appears to be used monotonously by certain elements of the pharmaceutical industry when they feel threatened by a competitor that is not under their control. Fortunately in this case, a judge ruled against the agency, so red-yeast extract can continue to be sold as a dietary supplement.

However, the following facts should be stated on the labels of all such medicines: RYE should not be combined with any other cholesterol- or lipid-lowering drugs; never take it with grapefruit juice, which can cause a build-up of lovastatin in the body, or with a large amount of niacin. To avoid possible complications caused by the statin in RYE, do not take the supplement if you are pregnant or breast-feeding, if you have liver disease, a serious infection or a transplanted organ, or if you have had recent major surgery.

INDIAN TERMINALIA
Terminalia arjuna

ASIA

For some 3,000 years, the valuable bark of the Arjuna tree, which is 80% soluble in water, has been used in Indian herbal medicine for heart conditions. Vagbhata, an Indian physican of the 7th century AD is reported to have been the first to prescribe arjuna for heart disease and it has been used in Ayurvedic practice for that purpose ever since.

In recent times, as with many other ancient remedies using medicinal plants, modern science is beginning to confirm what many herbal practitioners knew all along, but with the added advantage to being able to chemically analyze the plant's contents and also discover any contra-indications the plant may possess. The evaluation of this botanical medicine indicates that it can be of benefit in the treatment of coronary artery disease, heart failure and possibly hypercholesterolemia without adverse effects to the liver and renal functions, it also brings relief of anginal pain. In a large study of Arjuna administered to humans with coronary artery disease two patients with coronary heart failure showed significant improvement. It was found that prolonged use of Arjuna did not show any adverse effects on renal, hepatic and haematological parameters. In fact, the scientists who conducted the experiment recommended that the potential of Arjuna needs to be harnessed for coronary artery disease. More recent research also suggests that T. arjuna bark has significant antioxidant properties that are comparable with vitamin E and that it also has promising anti-carcinogenic potential.

8

Brain Power

Remember, it's thanks in part to Mum and her food fads during pregnancy that your brain is such a remarkable thing. It's the only one you will ever have, so it's going to be with you for life – brain transplants are not yet on the cards, let alone on the NHS. So important is this amazing organ that if someone is starving to death, as their body rapidly becomes emaciated, the weight of the brain and spinal cord hardly changes at all. The brain has two rich sources of energy in those unsaturated fatty acids, omega-3 and omega-6, of which it is made, but during starvation when they are in short supply, it can make use of breakdown products from other parts of the body as fuel.

Brains are extremely expensive things to have, for despite the fact that they make up only 2 per cent of our body mass, they consume 18 per cent of our energy budget. In a normal well fed human, glucose is the brain's chosen fuel. Unfortunately, animals – and that includes us – cannot make glucose from fatty acids; plants can, which is one reason, perhaps, that despite their lack of exercise we never see a fat plant.

As with our hearts, it is via the blood that our brains are kept supplied with all the glucose, minerals, vitamins, oxygen and unsaturated fat they need for constant rebuilding and repair. Two large arteries carry the blood up to the brain, and two main veins bring it back down to the heart. Spare a thought for giraffes next time you start to complain about headaches. Remember, too, that headaches are an important part of the body's early-warning system. They are in most cases not an illness in themselves, but simply a warning that something is wrong. All too often we treat the headache and not the cause, which is rather like turning off the alarm and leaving the burglar in the house.

Headaches are very common and can be caused by any number of factors including anxiety, stress, tension and hormonal disorders. They may come as an accompaniment to just about every disease or syndrome you may suffer from: even spinal misalignment, which starts with the skull, cranium and jaw – so if headaches persist a trip to the osteopath may help. Those with frequent headaches may have allergies to a whole variety of foodstuffs, especially additives. The best thing to do is to keep a record and check it out for yourself.

Migraine is a different kettle of fish, and may well signify that something is wrong with your brain itself, for the dilation of cranial blood vessels may be implicated. The difference between a migraine attack and an ordinary headache is that in the former the pain is often localised on one side of the head (though it may wander around to the other side and carry on with a second serving). It is also, more often than not, a throbbing rather than a steady pain. What is more, onset may be preceded by a characteristic feeling of ill-ease referred to as 'aura', and be accompanied by distortion of both vision and hearing, great sensitivity to light, nausea, vomiting, diarrhoea and even the kind of incapacity that requires total bed rest. Migraine is estimated to occur in about 10 per cent of the British population, and one survey found that 28 per cent of MPs suffered from it. Women suffer more than men do, so as the Houses of Parliament become better balanced genderwise, the figure may well go up.

Migraine may have a number of different clinical causes, but some forms are definitely food-related, in particular regarding those foods that are richest in amines and nitroamines such as cheese (especially blue), chocolate, citrus peel, red wine and, worst of all, port. For many people, low blood sugar caused by fasting (watch out, all you crash dieters!) or irregular meals often brings on a headache that quickly disappears after eating. But for people prone to migraines, the low-blood-sugar chain reaction is one that a belated meal will not stop.

Many researchers feel that serotonin, an important brain chemical and neurotransmitter, may fuel migraines. The platelets contain all of the serotonin normally present in blood; they aggregate when blood flow slows, releasing serotonin, which results in a potent constricting effect on the arteries.

Hangovers are a classic case of poisoning: the poisoning of our bodies with alcohol, a fuel on which you could run your car. Unfortunately, our bodies can't make direct use of alcohol even if it is five-star, so like all waste substances it gets carted round your body and dumped in your liver, ready to be dealt with. Too much alcohol and your liver, however well you may think you have trained it, becomes unable to cope and its poisoned cells die. Fortunately, our livers have remarkable powers of regeneration and do everything they can to repair the damage.

It is true that every one of us has a different capacity for alcohol, but a good rule of thumb is this: 'Two or three pints of beer two or three times a week – why spoil a good thing?' Well, that was the message I spelt out in a Health Education Council TV advert over two decades ago. The surprising thing was the number of letters I got saying, 'I wish I could afford nine pints a week and so follow your advice and stay healthy.' Facetious some comments undoubtedly were, but there was more than a grain of truth in them. The grain in question is barley, of course, another one of those all-important cereals. Think of all that stored energy made readily available and eminently digestible in the malting vat (the only good VAT I have ever come across), overflowing with minerals and vitamins thanks in part to brewer's yeast. Real ale is also a great diuretic, while hops are prescribed in herbal medicine as a remedy for anxiety and stress. Beer, especially organic real ale, could almost be a designer health food drink. Did you know that enlightened maternity units offer Guinness to pregnant mums? As with all good things, though, treat it with care, and always remember a pint of good ale contains as much alcohol as a double whisky.

FOOD FOR THOUGHT

Brain-building and -maintenance call for well protected bodywork and fuel for the engine from both food and drink. Burgers, hot-dogs, fried fish, bacon and eggs and, of course, French (despite the fact they were invented in Scotland) fries are not in themselves bad things. If they were, then the people of South-East Asia would be surprised at the increased stature of their children as they take on the fast-food way of life. But if the items just listed were all good things, local health authorities and insurance companies would not be planning for the increased costs in healthcare relating to heart attacks and strokes.

All these warnings about diet and heart attacks and so on also relate to strokes, for arteriosclerosis helps cause both. So, to rub it in again, our bodies need a regular supply of fatty acids – without them, we would die. Most of the fat will be used as a fuel to keep us going and growing when young, and going and in repair when old. Most of it will be burnt or, as we aren't dragons, oxidised, which is in effect one and the same process. No smoke or flames, just lots of waste heat that may help ward off hypothermia in winter. But the process puts a strain on the system, especially in summer, which is why regular exercise is so important to burn off the excess.

One thing that tends to muck it all up still further is the way we cook our food. Cooking is another form of oxidation: too much oxygen, and things burn too fast. That's where the smoke and flames come in, filling the kitchen. The nasty acrid stuff makes your eyes smart, and once inside you it does worse than that. The highly oxidised saturated fat in overdone food is toxic to the lining of your arteries, including those that keep your brain supplied. The brain isn't just a super virtual-reality computer capable of processing a mass of information, it is also our largest endocrine gland. This means that it produces hormones, the chemical messengers that oversee growth and development. In addition, one of its main jobs throughout evolution has been to help its owner avoid trouble, and that includes keeping him or her in good health.

Research is showing many links between the oldest and deepest part of the brain, the limbic system in which the hypothalamus sits, and the immune system. The latter, the body-wide system that helps protect us from most diseases, does its best even when challenged by AIDS. This prototype protection racket appears to work, at least in part, through those chemical messengers – including the brain's own brand – the endorphins, which have dealings with both pleasure and pain. A real Mafioso sort of relationship, for the endorphins, which are produced in the pituitary gland and stage-managed by the hypothalamus, are chemically akin to the opiates produced by the opium poppy.

A pin-prick hurts a lot, especially if anticipated, while a deep trauma, a cut or even a fracture, which are usually unexpected, are in comparison much less painful. The reason for this is that the brain comes to the rescue, pouring out its own brand of morphine. The brain can also convince us, after a mishap, that we feel better. There are many cases of soldiers suffering from really bad wounds, the kind that mean a ticket home, who have needed fewer pain-killers than those suffering from a minor injury. That's easy to understand, you might say. Well, how about cases of mock heart surgery in which the anaesthetised patient is opened up and closed again with all the trappings of surgery and convalescence, but without deep intervention – a procedure that has on occasion proved as effective as the complete operation. This must be looked upon as the ultimate placebo.

Impossible! you may say – there is no such thing as mind over matter! But I can remember as a child being dressed in my best clothes when taken to the doctor and being quite certain in advance that he was going to do me good – and I'm sure it made all the difference. Similarly, when I was ill I always felt better with Mum in charge; and once after a rugby accident (look at my nose), as soon as a St John Ambulance arrived on the scene. It's not just imagination; coming to your rescue is a crucially important function of your brain.

We hear a lot about Alzheimer's these days, and so we should, because it appears to be getting commoner. Some link it to the fact that we are living longer, and others to the increased use of novel chemicals in our modern lifestyles. This brain disorder usually occurs in the later years of life, although there are rare cases of it in younger people. Individuals with Alzheimer's disease develop progressive loss of memory and gradually lose the ability to function and to take care of themselves. The cause of this disorder is not known. Some studies suggest that it may be related to an accumulation of aluminium in the brain, yet aluminium toxicity has been studied in humans and is quite distinct from Alzheimer's. So this remains an unresolved issue.

Aluminium is one of the commonest elements on the face of the earth; in fact, we live from the crumbs that fall from the earth's crust, which is made mainly of slightly acidic aluminium silicate. Fortunately for life and for us, aluminium, which is highly toxic, is insoluble at the normal range of acidity found upon the earth's surface.

Preliminary evidence has linked populations at high risk from Alzheimer's disease with higher levels of dietary fat and calories; similarly, fish intake has been linked with low-risk populations. Highly antioxidant foods, when incorporated into the everyday diet, are considered to reduce the risk of Alzheimer's. The most important are those with large amounts of vitamins E and C, carotenes – especially beta-carotene – and the metal selenium. There is also a growing body of evidence indicating that recent changes in diet may be implicated. Fish on Friday, with a supper of cod, haddock or rock salmon to round off a hard working week, was evidently a brainy idea. And kippers or poached haddock for breakfast, roe on toast, bloaters, mackerel, jellied eels, selenium-rich shellfish such as shrimps and prawns, whelks, winkles and even clams (all good sources of omega-3 fatty acids) for tea were facts of my childhood diet. As late as the nineteenth century, oysters were staple sources of protein for those urban poor who lived near an estuary and, in the days of clean rivers, salmon runs were so abundant that the dead salmon were used as a fertiliser.

Fish has long been considered as 'brain food', and recent work summarised by Dr Norman Salem at the US National Institute of Mental Health proves the point. Many detailed studies show that low levels of the omega-3 fatty acids, especially one fraction called DHA (a rich source of which is salmon), are linked to depression, aggressive behaviour, brain damage from alcohol, attention deficit disorder (ADD) and possibly Alzheimer's disease. Salem explains that DHA fatty acid helps regulate the cell membrane functions involved in transmitting signals among brain cells. Research suggests that it's easier for brain chemicals such as serotonin to transmit messages when the consistency of the fat in the membranes surrounding the brain cells is fluid and flexible, like fish oil, rather than hardened stuff like lard. If you don't feed brain-cell membranes enough of the right type of fat, the messages may be short-circuited and garbled.

SIBERIAN GINSENG
Eleutherococcus senticosus
ASIA

Siberian ginseng, or eleuthero, is a native of the taiga region of Siberia, south-east Russia, northern China, Korea and Japan. Although not as popular as Asian ginseng, both the roots and the rhizomes of Siberian ginseng are popular in the West. According to Chinese medicine records, the use of eleuthero dates back two thousand years; referred to as *ci wu ju*, it was used to prevent respiratory-tract infections as well as colds and flu. People in the Siberian taiga region used to find that it increased stamina and decreased the incidence of infections.

Explorers, divers, sailors and miners used it to prevent stress-related illness.

Eleuthero does indeed increase energy and stamina, and helps people to resist and relieve physical stress more effectively, as well as alleviating headache and insomnia, and increasing mental alertness without the let-down that comes with caffeinated products. In more modern times, eleuthero's ability to increase endurance has led Soviet Olympic athletes to use it to enhance their training.

Russian research since the 1950s has shown that eleuthero is a stimulant, that it normalises arterial pressure, mediates against hardening of the arteries and angina, improves blood circulation and reduces elevated blood-sugar and cholesterol levels. As an 'adaptogen', it helps the body to cope by encouraging the adrenal glands to function optimally when challenged by stress. Contemporary Australian research suggests it may act as a 'stress modulator' – that is, below a certain threshold it increases the stress response and above that threshold it decreases the stress response.

One German laboratory study has demonstrated that eleuthero extract inhibits the replication of all ribonucleic viruses studied so far as well as inhibiting the replication of the human rhinovirus, which causes respiratory infections in man, and that it possesses the ability to support the immune system. Originating in the cold steppes of Russia, Siberian ginseng is at last having its scientific colours nailed to the mast. That long-awaited step has finally been taken towards the acceptance of the herbal cornucopia as the source of remedies for our common ills and as a bulwark against them.

KAVA
Piper methysticum
PACIFIC ISLANDS

'Have a bilo of yaqona!' (*Mai dua na bilo!*) Bring some sunshine into your stressed existence! You will be in the good and healthy company of the Pacific royal families, for yaqona, better known as kava, is Fiji's national drink. Kava is a member of the pepper family and grows as a bush in the South Pacific islands. It was on Captain James Cook's voyage of 1768–71 that Europeans first encountered the plant at sacred ceremonies and named it 'intoxicating pepper'. The precise origins of Oceanic kava are not certain because the Pacific Islands had an oral tradition, not a written one. However, using botanical evidence, ethno botanist Vincent Lebot's idea that kava originated somewhere in Melanesia, either on Vanuatu, the Solomon Islands or New Guinea, seems probable. Whatever its origins, kava has been used for over three thousand years among the peoples of the Pacific Islands, both in ceremonies and for medicinal purposes. Today, this traditional drink still plays a key role in Vanuatuan, Fijian, Samoan and Tongan societies and continues to be used to honour visitors, unite participants in key ceremonies and validate their social identities. Recent research suggests that, given the low incidence of cancer in kava-consuming populations such as Vanuatu and Fiji, there is a close inverse relationship between the disease and kava consumption.

A soothing drink with scientifically proven medicinal effects, kava is an excellent herb for calming the nerves and easing stress, while combating fatigue in a natural way. Its antidepressant components fight the 'blues' and induce tranquillity. Kava promotes deep and restful sleep, and is particularly useful for treating ailments such as migraine, headaches and cramps, offering the added advantage of keeping the mind alert while relaxing the body.

Components including lactones have been isolated from the kava rhizome, many of which are known to be psychoactive. Kava appears to act on the brain's limbic system, which governs basic responses such as 'fright or flight'. It has been tested for use in controlling anxiety, with good results. It may also provide an excellent therapeutic tool for the treatment of women suffering from anxiety and depression during the menopause. Kava therapy accelerates the resolution of psychological symptoms without diminishing the therapeutic action of oestrogens being taken for problems such as osteoporosis and cardiovascular disease.

Kava has a direct effect on muscle tension similar to that of ordinary tranquillisers. The herb has also been shown to be antioxidant and to protect the brain during periods of low blood flow. This has led to speculation that it may be useful as a pre-anaesthetic treatment for patients before operations. However, if kava or any other herbal remedies, whether prescribed or self-administered, are being taken, this must be reported before any operation is performed, as kava compounds have been found to interfere with anaesthesia. Experiences related amongst the Pacific Islanders and the Aborigines of Australia have indicated that, if taken to excess, kava has a stupor-inducing narcotic effect. It is not recommended for those who suffer from liver complaints or are taking hepatic medication, or where quick reaction time is required, such as when driving. Kava is also contra-indicated for use by pregnant and lactating women; by those suffering from Parkinson's disease or using anti-anxiety agents such as antidepressants, antipsychotics or other agents causing depression; by those using sedatives or hypnotics; or for undiagnosed types of depression. And it should not be taken with alcohol or barbiturates. The list is long and getting longer, as the fors and againsts are locked in battle over the rights and wrongs of short-term profit. Recently Kava Kava has been withdrawn from open sale in Australia and the UK.

MAIDEN HAIR TREE
Ginkgo biloba
CHINA

Once a food plant of the dinosaurs and first known only as a fossil, this strange tree was found in cultivation around temples in China and more recently growing wild as a forest tree in the Himalayas. Its yellow fruits are eaten to this day. Medicinal use of ginkgo can be traced back almost five thousand years in Chinese herbal medicine. It was recommended for respiratory-tract ailments as well as memory loss in the elderly. *Ginkgo biloba* extract has long been popular in Europe and elsewhere for its neuroprotective properties.

The main thrust of present scientific investigation has concentrated on the plant's leaves and the active constituents ginkgolides and bilobalide, chemicals unknown in any other plant species. Ginkgolides may improve circulation and inhibit the platelet-activating factor which in large amounts is associated with nerve-cell damage and poor blood flow to the central nervous system. Extracts of the plant's leaves have been shown to stimulate the flow of blood to the deepest parts of the brain, to protect the brain from the ingress of poisons and enhance the processing of information by the nerve cells. Among other things, ginkgo shows promise in the treatment of dementia and other manifestations of ageing. Over four hundred scientific studies have established the importance of ginkgo in improving poor cerebral circulation, aiding memory and concentration and helping in cases of mild cognitive impairment in the elderly. It can also help to prevent altitude sickness. Indeed, *Ginkgo biloba* is currently one of the most extensively studied and most widely used substances for improving cognition and enhancing the activities of daily living.

If you are using ginkgo and are about to have an operation, tell your GP and any other physicians concerned. Ginkgo should be used cautiously, or avoided altogether, by anyone predisposed to seizure or using other medicines known to incite seizure. It should not be taken with anticoagulant, anti-platelet agents, tricyclic antidepressants or anticonvulsants. In rare instances, sensitive individuals may get a rash after taking *Ginkgo biloba* supplement, but this is due more to an excess of the allergen ginkgolic acid produced during manufacture.

Research into ginkgo is ongoing, and it is to be hoped that further research will reveal more aids to human health. The health-giving properties of ginkgo are so highly regarded in the South Korean capital Seoul that 200 kilogrammes of the fruit are collected annually from urban trees and used in social welfare programmes.

WILLOWS
Salix spp.

Willow bark has been used to alleviate the pain of headaches since time immemorial. Found to contain an algesic, salicylic acid, it 'green'-printed the worlds first synthetic pain killer: aspirin. Willow was used by the ancient Egyptians to treat inflammation, while Hippocrates recommended chewing willow leaves for women in labour. Traditionally, astringent White Willow [Salix alba] extract was used to staunch internal bleeding and the bark extract has been used as an alternative medicine for low back pain since Dioscorides first recorded it in the 1st century AD.

Clinical research began in earnest in the early 1800's (it was first synthesized in 1838) and by the turn of the 19th century asprin had gained worldwide recognition in the treatment of pain and rheumatological disorders. Reports on adverse events relating to gastrointestinal intolerance and bleeding appeared early, but were largely neglected until the 1950s.

Sir John Vane elucidated aspirin's active mechanism as an inhibitor of prostaglandin synthetase and received the Nobel Prize in Medicine for this work in 1982. Now, after two centuries of evaluation, aspirin remains topical and new therapeutic uses are still being found and studied. This is also true of White Willow itself, which, unlike asprin does not thin the blood. Nor does it irritate the stomach lining, which is a common side effect of aspirin. Recently, an expert committee on herbal remedies established by Germany's Federal Institute for Drugs and Medical Devices has approved White willow bark as an herb that can be used to treat pain and inflammation associated with headaches.

Recent studies of willow bark extract use in America and Germany indicate that not only is the extract very successful in dealing with acute lower back pain, as history relates, but it offers a very real economic impact on the cost of treatment for this condition. Willow should not be taken with prescribed anticoagulant drugs. As I dot the I's and cross the T's on these final page proofs good news comes in from Cumbria, 'Lakeland Willow Water' from a spring naturally enriched with salicin forms the basis of what is already a big business. Salicin, like its synthetic counterpart Asprin is already proving successful in the prevention of deep vein thrombosis and in lowering the risk of heart attack and strokes. It may well prove that this water needs no artificial fizz.

9

You and Your Hormones

There is no getting away from the fact that we are what we eat, but from that point on our hormones take over.

Hormones are made from lipids and are produced by your endocrine glands. Starting at the top, the pineal gland is situated between the two hemispheres of the brain. Research tells us that the pineal is all we have left of a third eye, which used to look upwards. Pineal hormones control your circadian rhythm: your reactions to your own internal clock that is set at a cycle of around twenty-four hours. 'Are you a late-night person or an early-morning person?' – I reckon this should be a compulsory question when it comes to marriage guidance. Also, how do you each react to jetlag? I always say it has little effect on me, but my family says that I am permanently in that state of halfway from somewhere.

The hypothalamus, that oldest and deepest part of the brain, makes hormones that may help sperms on their way by causing uterine contraction during sexual stimulation, as well as other hormones that control the body's water balance and stimulate the nearby pituitary gland to release *its* hormones.

Your pituitary gland is located at the base of your brain, at the level of your tonsils (if you've still got them; I hope you have because they are an important part of your lymphatic system – mine were whipped out before their importance was understood). That's about the safest, most protected, location in the whole of your body – the perfect place for the gland that masterminds the production of sex hormones, controls sperm, egg and milk production and stimulates other glands to release their own hormones.

Your thyroid is the governor within you. Situated in your neck, it makes thyroxine, which affects the rate of your body processes including heat production, energy release from food, and the growth and development of your nervous system. Separate, but part of your thyroid, the parathyroids control the amount of calcium in your blood and bones. Iodine is very important in the working of the thyroid, and populations living a long way from the sea (which produces most of our iodine-rich foods) were often found to suffer from goitre (the symptoms of which were large swellings of the neck) until iodine was added to the salt cellar.

Sitting on top of your kidneys, not a nice place to get kicked in, your adrenal glands produce a range of hormones which help you deal with stress, control water balance and oversee the development of gender features at puberty and thereafter. They also produce adrenaline – the trigger to your personal emergency services that make you get up and go. You know that all-over feeling: your face goes pale as blood is diverted to your muscles from skin and gut; your liver pours out energy-rich food; your spleen releases extra blood corpuscles to carry oxygen. You breathe faster, your heart speeds up and you go into a cold sweat, cooling those muscles that are making your escape – you hope. What is more, if trauma results your blood clots faster to heal the wound.

A small organ below your stomach, the pancreas, secretes 'juice' containing carbohydrate, protein and fat-splitting enzymes, into the duodenum, an organ that greatly aids the digestion of food. The pancreas also releases the hormone insulin into the bloodstream, where it helps control blood-sugar levels by commanding your muscles to store it away ready for use as the need arises and as adrenaline commands.

Last but not least, your testes or ovarian follicles are also in the hormone business. The former make testosterone, which determines all your male characteristics and aspirations. The ovarian follicles make oestrogen, and that is why girls will be girls, women will be women and mums will be mums. The role of the sex hormones during childhood is still shrouded in mystery. It is your brain that turns you on at puberty by telling your pituitary to increase the production of hormones, which stir testes and ovaries into action.

Hormones are wonderful things, and they are all made from cholesterol, one reason why our bodies have a love–hate relationship with the stuff.

PSEUDO-GINSENG
Panax notoginseng
CHINA

Pseudo-ginseng, or *san qi*, is cultivated in many provinces of southern and central China, but is fast becoming extinct in the wild. *San qi* is a traditional tonic that supports the function of the adrenal glands, in particular the production of male sex hormones and corticosteroids (the steroids that are normally produced by your adrenal glands). In computer-assisted semen-analysis evaluation, *san qi* extracts have been seen to improve motility in both normal and inferior sperm. Pseudo-gingseng's chemical make-up permits it to normalise heart rate, blood pressure and circulation, and it helps to prevent fatigue and relieve stress. The herb also reduces inflammation and relieves pain, and has bactericidal properties. Western practitioners involved with sports frequently give it as a tonic to improve stamina.

American and Chinese scientific research has confirmed *san qi*'s established reputation as a means of arresting bleeding. However, unlike Western medications, the root once described as 'more valuable than gold' seems to halt bleeding *without* making the blood clot, and to stop the clotting or the haematoma without causing bleeding. Notoginseng is among those herbs that Chinese scientists think may be beneficial in the treatment of inadequate blood flow to the brain, and there is increasing evidence that it enhances cognition.

KELPS AND WRACKS
Laminaria spp., Fucus spp.
TEMPERATE SEAS

Those large brown seaweeds washed up on the beach have been used for centuries as a rich source of natural organic minerals and vitamins. Earliest records, from 3000 BC, indicate that in China the Emperor Shen-neng used seaweeds as both medicine and food. In Japan today seaweeds form up to 25 per cent of the diet and are generally seen as keeping at bay disease, fat and the deterioration caused by ageing. Dietary seaweed is also credited with being part of the reason why Japan has a lower incidence of breast cancer, constipation and gastrointestinal ailments than other countries.

Kelp contains over sixty elements, twenty-one amino acids and thirteen vitamins, and is the only known vegetable source of vitamin B_{12}. It is especially rich in iodine, calcium, sulphur and silicon. Kelp's high trace-mineral content helps to regulate the secretion of hormones. In particular, its high iodine content is beneficial to the thyroid and the liver, and activates and regulates the metabolism – which is why it is seen as a general tonic. Kelp can also help to burn off excess fat and so protect against atherosclerosis and obesity. To avoid the interference of the iodine contained in kelp with prescribed thyroid hormones, do not take kelp at the same time; and don't take it with warfarin either, because of the otherwise beneficial high vitamin K content in kelp.

The properties of seaweed are seemingly limitless and are being researched around the world. In Germany it was recently found that bladderwrack (*Fucus vesiculosus*) is active against HIV.

LIQUORICE
Glycyrrhiza glabra
EUROPE

Liquorice is cultivated throughout Europe, the Middle East and Asia, and is one of the most popular and widely consumed herbs in the world. The medicinal use of liquorice in both Western and Eastern cultures dates back several thousand years. The first recorded medicinal use was discovered on Assryian clay tablets (c. 2500 BC). Wild liquorice was used by native North Americans for childbirth problems and menstruation. It is the second most prescribed herb in China today, where it has been used for over two thousand years as a tonic to rejuvenate the heart and spleen. Called *gancao* in China, it is also used there to improve liver function in patients suffering from hepatitis and to clear jaundice. It is a rising star of Japanese research in helping to treat cases of chronic hepatitis C, for which there is no known cure. The most common medicinal use for liquorice is still in the treatment of upper respiratory ailments such as coughs, hoarseness, sore throat and bronchitis. It is also important for the treatment of stomach and intestinal ulcers.

Liquorice has a marked effect upon the endocrine system, encouraging the production of hormones such as hydrocortisone which have anti-inflammatory properties, and it reduces the breakdown of steroids by the liver and kidneys. Its anti-inflammatory action also plays a role in stimulating the adrenal cortex, and it is often used following steroid therapy. Like cortisone, it can relieve arthritic and allergy symptoms, but without side-effects. It has proven useful in treating menopausal symptoms, regulating menstruation and relieving menstrual cramps, and may be used by women to stabilise the menstrual cycle when coming off 'the pill'. Be aware before using liquorice, if you are taking prescribed corticosteroid drugs or the immunosuppressant cyclosporin, that the herb may intensify their effect or interfere with their mechanisms. Such drugs include the diuretic spirono-lactone, thiazide diuretics, cardiac glycosides and monoamine oxidase inhibitors (MAOIs). Problems with liquorice can be largely avoided by using a deglycyrrhizinated preparation.

ASPARAGUS
Asparagus officinalis
EURASIA, NORTH AFRICA

Asparagus is claimed to increase feelings of compassion and love and to be an aphrodisiac. In fact, this plant has been associated over the centuries with almost all aspects of hormones and hormone production. Like garlic, no sooner have you eaten it than it is pouring from your skin a distillate that turns others either on or off. Although these days asparagus is mainly valued as an exotic food, it has long been used in medicine. There are ancient Egyptian tomb drawings of it from c. 4000 BC, and indications that it was used for urinary conditions and for worming. During the Renaissance, asparagus was promoted as an aphrodisiac and banned from the tables of most nunneries. A sixteenth-century Arabian love manual contained an asparagus recipe, and in eighteenth-century France the notorious Madame de Pompadour used asparagus for sexual vigour. Being in good health has a lot to do with libido. Asparagus is a nourishing, blood-building tonic that enhances the health of both male and female reproductive organs.

In India another species, *A. racemosus*, is used to increase sperm count and to nourish the ovum. In Ayurvedic medicine it is a very important herb for women – its Ayurvedic name, *shatavari*, means 'she who has one hundred husbands'. It has now been found that asparagus root contains compounds called steroid glycosides, which directly affect hormone production and may very well influence the more primitive emotions.

In the West asparagus has been shown to help rid the body of excess water and salt, and to help prevent anaemia caused by folic acid deficiency. Used topically, it soothes the pain and swelling of joints due to rheumatism or arthritis, and is used to alleviate the pain of kidney-stones. In modern Germany, the root appears in diuretic 'water pill' preparations, as well as in formulas for urinary-tract inflammation and infection and kidney-stone prevention. Most recent research is looking into the adaptogenic potential of the herb. The sometimes malodorous effect on urine from eating asparagus is harmless, and probably due to its sulphur content.

TURMERIC
Curcuma longa
SOUTHERN ASIA

A key ingredient of curry powder, turmeric is extensively cultivated in all parts of India, but particularly in Madras, Bengal and Bombay. It is also cultivated in southern mainland China, Taiwan, Japan, Burma, Indonesia and throughout the African continent.

Turmeric is a herb of major importance in the East, and in recent times has received more attention in the West. The Chinese use it against numerous intestinal infections and ailments. In India, it is used for digestive, circulatory and respiratory complaints. Turmeric works well against bacteria to do with the spoilage of food, as well as fighting the infection of wounds. It shows promise in preventing the damage caused to the liver by alcohol and by certain pharmaceutical drugs, especially acetaminophen in high doses. Research has shown turmeric to have many useful properties, particularly in the anti-inflammatory and anti-hepato-toxic range.

The herb has been investigated for its influence on the secretion of bile and pancreatic and gastric juices. It has been found to increase bile flow and to protect the stomach and liver from a number of toxic compounds. And because it stimulates the flow of bile, it aids the digestion of fat.

The active agent, curcumin, has a wide range of therapeutic effects. It is a strong antioxidant, reduces inflammation and histamine levels, and may increase the production of natural cortisone by the adrenal glands. Its anti-inflammatory effect is even stronger than that of hydrocortisone, and is comparable in potency to that of the non-steroidal phenylbutazone. In recent animal research into the antioxidant protection of neuronal pathways in Alzheimer's disease, it has been shown that, whereas vitamin E even in high concentration is unable to protect cells from oxidation, the curcuminoids in turmeric are highly antioxidant. Curcumin is also antibacterial, and lowers cholesterol levels. It has a contraceptive effect in rats, is antibiotic, and has proved antiprotozoal in vitro. A small amount of turmeric is used in numerous multi-ingredient remedies that help regulate the flow of bile.

With all this good research now in the public domain, it was little wonder that an American doctor tried to patent the virtues of turmeric as a drug. Thank goodness this attempt was thrown out by the court, thus preserving the rights of everyone in the world to derive the many benefits of the age-old tradition of this food medicine.

A few people are allergic to turmeric, and should not continue to take it if they experience breathing problems or tightness in the throat or chest, chest pain, hives or other rashes, or itchy, swollen skin.

MACA
Lepidium meyenii
SOUTH AMERICA

Maca is a pear-shaped tuberous root that grows in the Andes on some of the harshest farmlands in the world. It was cultivated by Inca farmers for food and medicine nearly three thousand years ago. Highly valued as a nutritious food by native Peruvians, it was used as an energiser, an aphrodisiac and for fertility, and against impotence. Hence it was dubbed 'Peruvian ginseng'. Grown in the Peruvian altiplano, maca is used to improve the libido of both men and women. It has also been used for many other ailments including tuberculosis and anaemia, and by women during the menopause.

Weight-lifters and body-builders are turning to maca as a natural and safe alternative to anabolic steroids. The herb is considered to be adaptogenic, helping to restore balance to the body. Unlike caffeine, maca is not a stimulant, and can be used to enhance both physical and mental energy. A single dried maca root contains almost 60 phytochemicals, 18 amino acids, 7 minerals including iodine, 6 plant sterols and 20 fatty acids; and it comes with a full array of vitamins as well as saponins, tannins and other active compounds. It is still used for problems to do with the menopause, and for pre-menstrual syndrome. Its calcium and magnesium content and its alkaloids benefit the female endocrine system, and the iodine in it benefits the thyroid.

Maca's fertility-enhancing properties have been endorsed since 1961, when research demonstrated that it increased fertility in rats. It is now known that its effects in humans are not limited to the ovaries and testes: it also acts on the pancreas and thyroid, as well as on the adrenals, giving a feeling of greater energy and vitality. This superfood of the Incas is one of the best natural invigorating and revitalising substances, helping to overcome energy loss and the wear and tear caused by our accelerated lifestyles and poor nutrition.

PATA DE VACA, COW'S HOOF
Bauhinia forficata
SOUTH AMERICA

Pata de vaca, so called because the shape of its leaf resembles a cow's hoof, is a rainforest treasure whose appreciation by the West has perhaps come just in time to help in the fight against diabetes, which is rapidly gaining almost epidemic proportions on this side of the planet. It is a modern legend of Brazilian herbalism, originating in 1950 when one Friar Luíz Maria set off to find a Dr Christophe in the campo grande, seeking – and finding – a cure for his diabetes. The good doctor had learned the use of this herb, traditionally applied by the local forest dwellers and farmers for elephantiasis, snakebite and all manner of skin problems.

The Peruvians consider *pata de vaca* to be a detoxifying herb helping to combat impurity in the blood and organs and to alleviate low blood pressure; and a diuretic useful for renal and urinary problems such as the overproduction of urine. In South America it is an esteemed treatment for diabetes, taking the nickname 'vegetable Insulin', having been used for over sixty years to balance blood-sugar levels in diabetics. The herb contains flavonoids, glycosides, saponins, tannins and other agents, and is a 'teabag treatment', readily available to the general public, to be drunk after meals.

The beneficial effects of *pata de vaca* on hypoglycaemia were first reported in a clinical study in 1929. In 1945 clinicians attempted unsuccessfully to determine the active constituents that caused such effects. Lack of funding for research into non-proprietary drugs did not stop the locals, who knew they were on to a good thing, and over many years they provided practical evidence of the herb's prowess. However, it was not until the mid-

1980s, with *pata*'s continued use as an insulin substitute combined with a much wider public interest in complementary medicine, that further research was begun. It is to be hoped that this 'natural plant insulin', which has already left its hoof prints in the sands of time, will now receive the positive scientific attention it deserves to back up its popular use.

QUORN
Fusarium graminearum
BRITAIN

A remarkable late-twentieth-century discovery, this tiny fungus was found growing in a field in Buckinghamshire in the early 1960s. Found to be a cholesterol-free and fibre-rich source of non-meat protein, it is now grown in continuous culture and is processed into nutritious 'steaks' suitable for vegetarians. Research is going on apace and preliminary results suggest it might be of use in the treatment of diabetes, helping to sate the diabetic patient and so reduce the amount of food consumed (especially useful in the evening).

10

Dem Bones

All two hundred and six of them. Very few of our bones are actually connected directly to each other, whatever the song may suggest, but they are interlinked at the joints by tough ligaments. Bones are made of two sorts of material: minerals and collagen. Minerals, mainly calcium phosphate and calcium carbonate, give them strength and rigidity. The latter is the stuff the white cliffs of Dover are made of – in fact, those cliffs are the fossilised skeletons of tiny sea creatures. If you give a bone the acid-bath treatment it keeps its shape but becomes flexible. This flexibility is thanks mainly to the other component, collagen, the structural protein that gives it strength. Destroy the protein by heating in an oven, and the bone becomes very brittle as the organic material is burned away.

Under normal circumstances, like all the other parts of your body the bones are kept in good repair all the time and, if treated in the right way, heal remarkably quickly. However, once you are past forty years of age, healing and repair take longer. Back in the bad old days of the Industrial Revolution when diets were as poor as the living conditions in the dark tenement blocks, rickets was a common problem, and children with bowed legs and other malformed bones a common sight.

Rickets was eventually shown to be linked to lack of exposure to sunshine, which produces vitamin D_3 in the skin by its action on dehydroxycholesterol. (That stuff gets everywhere.) Today the main bone complaint and the main cure are osteoporosis and hip/knee/shoulder etc. replacement. (The former is nothing new, for it was common in Egyptian mummies.) Osteoporosis appears to be a speeding-up of the normal degenerative processes of old age in which both of the main bone constituents diminish. Some links have been found with a high-phosphate, low-calcium diet; and research goes on apace, with over fifteen million people in the USA alone suffering from the complaint.

Only ten years ago, osteoporosis was usually dismissed as a normal part of ageing. The National Osteoporosis Society has recently done a fine job in campaigning to change the medical profession's understanding of the disease. Most GPs and practice nurses are now very aware of how much can be done to prevent and treat osteoporosis successfully. There's a great deal that people can effectively do for themselves, and the experts at the NOS are happy to offer advice and support if you need it.

The following statistics and advice are adapted from their leaflet *Fighting Fragile Bones*:

* 'You are sure to know someone, maybe a relative, with osteoporosis because it is now a serious epidemic in Britain. One in three women and one in twelve men over fifty in the UK are at risk of suffering painful and deforming fractures as a result of osteoporosis. Every three minutes someone in the UK fractures a bone because of osteoporosis. Patients who have it fill a third of the orthopaedic beds in our hospitals. It is costing the country over £750 million each year and that is a conservative estimate (even under New Labour). More women die after hip fractures than from cancer of the ovaries, cervix and uterus.'
 * 'By early next century there could be five million sufferers in Britain unless we take major action now.'

The good news is that you can avoid osteoporosis.

* 'If you already have it, it can probably be treated and further bone loss prevented, so act now! At or after the menopause see your GP or practice nurse. There may be a clinic you can attend for menopause and osteoporosis therapy advice.'

As coffee, alcohol and smoking all appear to increase the likelihood of the disease – indeed, smokers have a 15–30 per cent lower bone-mineral content than non-smokers – a key part of that advice is to gradually change your lifestyle.

CASING YOUR JOINTS

Your body contains three main sorts of joints: fibrous, which allow no movement; cartilaginous, which allow only a little movement; and synovial, which give us freedom of movement and can cause us trouble. All of them contain a lot of the structural protein, collagen.

Synovial joints come in six sorts:

* ball-and-socket (also known as an enarthrosis), e.g. hip
* hinge (also known as a ginglymus), e.g. elbow, knee
* saddle, e.g. thumb
* condyloid, e.g. between lower jaw and skull
* pivot (also known as a trochoid), e.g. neck
* gliding, e.g. wrist

Go on, now give them a good gentle work-out, wave them about a bit – and whether you get a twinge or not, read on.

Synovial joints are encased within a fibrous capsule; the ends of the bones are covered with smooth cartilage so that they can slide over each other, and are lubricated by a fluid produced by the synovial membrane. This is a really sophisticated bit of self-lubricating independent suspension, which is subject to a great deal of wear and tear and can be damaged by accident, injury and, of course, substance abuse. Alcohol and tobacco are included here, but also too much food, for the heavier you are the more your joints are going to suffer.

Gout is not just a disease of florid old men – as I mentioned earlier, it can strike at any time, and it hurts. The pain is caused by crystals of uric acid, a natural waste product of our bodies, being dumped in our joints. Knuckles, toes and finger joints, which often do little work and so have a poor blood supply, are usually the first to be affected. Alcohol and aspirin may relieve the pain in the short term but they can aggravate the condition, the latter by inhibiting the secretion of uric acid. The main problem appears to be an inability of the kidneys to get rid of this waste product as nature intended.

Arthritis comes in two forms:

* *osteoarthritis* is unfortunately a degenerative disease of the joints, which can gradually creep up on us in old age. Around

85 per cent of people over seventy are afflicted, and under the age of forty-five, men are most likely to get it. Those smooth cartilages begin to degrade and so don't slide about as easily as they used to, while calcified osteophytes (even the name hurts), little spurs of limestone, develop on the joint margins. (This is why people don't complain about hip replacements, only about what caused them.)

* *rheumatoid arthritis* is a chronic joint disease and can strike at any time, causing many of the same symptoms and problems.

Weight-watching and regular gentle exercise, walking, tea dances and t'ai chi, can and do work wonders, by keeping all those joints on the move. A very recent development in Britain has been the setting up of 'green gyms', where a whole range of mentally and physically stressed people come and work out. 'Work out' is the operative term, for they go out and about in the community, planting trees, tending urban green space, helping in woodland management and even building dry-stone walls. The results in social and physical improvement for many must be seen to be believed.

Did you know that you are longer when you wake up in the morning than you were when you went to bed? Back in medieval times the French peasantry knew all about this, for recruits who wanted to get accepted into the army always presented themselves in the early morning when they could be as much as 1.6 centimetres taller. The Vicar of Aynho in Northamptonshire was the first to measure the difference (although he did it in twelfthimals) back in 1724. As he could find no such changes when he measured his horse, he concluded that it must be due to compression of the vertebral column, at least in adult humans. Children and adolescents do actually grow at night, when growth hormones are secreted in a series of pulses. These act through several intermediary stages to cause lengthening of the bones at the end-plates. Then, once growth has ceased, our nightly changes in stature are indeed due, at least in part, to the relaxing of those inter-vertebral discs when we lie down.

While your brain is protected by a bony case called a skull, the rest of your central nervous system, your spinal chord, is protected by the series of bones that it runs through called (as you know) vertebrae – and we all know what happens if that gets broken. To allow flexibility and movement, discs made of cartilage are strategically located in between each pair of vertebrae. It is the force of gravity acting on your weight that compresses the discs during the day, accounting for around 20 per cent of that daily loss of length. The other 80 per cent is due to your kyphosis and lordosis – the curves in your backbone, or your deportment. These curves vary with body weight (watch it!) and position. No wonder those uncompacted discs are wont to slip as we throw our full weight on them after a good night's sleep.

Weight-watching, regular whole-body exercise and common sense when lifting heavy things are without doubt the best way to avoid back trouble. Swimming can be very beneficial, as the water takes the weight off your discs and curves allowing all-over exercise to get to work. My mum took to the water in her seventies and never looked back. A warning to all grandfathers-to-be: watch it, babies and especially toddlers are very awkward things to pick up – always bend your knees and keep a straight back. Why not join your daughter or daughter-in-law in her pre-parenthood exercises, including those relating to relaxation? You're going to need it.

WINTERGREEN
Gaultheria procumbens
NEW WORLD

With a smell that conjures up images of sweaty locker rooms, wintergreen oil is used chiefly as an ointment or liniment for rheumatism. It was named after Jean-François Gaulthier (1708–56), a physician and botanist working in Canada. Today this and many other *Gaultheria* species are used as garden plants, prized for their waxy white or pink bell-shaped flowers, brilliant red fruits and orderly habit. The Inuit people of Labrador eat the berries raw and use the leaves to treat aching muscles, headache and sore throat. Elsewhere the herb is used mainly for joints and for muscular and nerve problems causing pain, such as lumbago. As well as for rheumatism, it is used for sciatica, a neurological condition where pain is caused by pressure on a nerve in the lower spine, trigeminal neuralgic pain which affects a facial nerve, and sprains and arthritis. The astringent oil is mildly analgesic, strongly anti-inflammatory, antiseptic, stimulant and diuretic. Wintergreen oil contains about 98 per cent methyl salicylate which has a similar effect to aspirin and most of which is now synthesised. True wintergreen oil is almost obsolete.

It is advisable to purchase proprietary ointments or salves containing wintergreen as the oil has been found to be toxic, irritant and sensitising, especially in those sensitive to aspirin.

CELERY
Apium graveolens
EUROPE

When it comes to the crunch, celery is one of those common salad plants we all take for granted and is much loved by Europeans and Asians alike. It was first used medicinally in ancient Egypt for various ills: for example, to cool the uterus and as a remedy for a painful stomach or swollen limbs. Even in those days its calcium content was tacitly recognised as a remedy for treating and fixing teeth. In the West, the German monk and poet Valafriedus Strabus first documented its use in the ninth century. In medical herbalism, as a remedy for arthritis and rheumatism, celery seeds are employed to help the kidneys dispose of urates, to reduce acidity in the body generally, to detoxify, and to improve circulation to the muscles and joints.

Research has found that celery stimulates urine production and has a flushing effect that helps to prevent the build-up of excess uric acid forming as crystals in the joints. This is related to fluid retention in the body and is the root of much joint pain in rheumatic, arthritic and gout sufferers. Celery contains carotene and vitamin B complex, E and C in small amounts and minerals including selenium, plus an anti-inflammatory agent. Many studies have shown that a vegetarian diet can help relieve rheumatoid arthritis, and anti-inflammatory celery is part of that regime.

Unfortunately, some people are allergic to celery and to the entire carrot, or Umbelliferae, family of herbs, vegetables and spices. However, German researchers are investigating a method of dealing with this hypersensitisation, using natural celery juice. But don't try it at home – it must be administered under strict supervision.

STINGING NETTLE
Urtica spp.

Used cooked as a nutrient-rich spring vegetable, nettles are found across the world, usually growing in soils rich in phosphates. Across the millennia, the strong stem fibres have been used to make fishing nets (hence their common name) and lines, and woven as cloth. The Romans used the nettle for curative flagellation in the cold climate of Britain, and to this day stories of miraculous cures relate to contact with the stinging hairs that cover the leaves and stems.

Research in 1991 confirms that the persistence of the stinging sensation experienced on contact with the leaf or stem may be caused by substances in the nettle fluid that are toxic to nerves or that trigger the release of other substances. Five years later further research considered that the action of the leaves might explain the positive effects of this extract in the treatment of rheumatic diseases. More recent research at Plymouth Postgraduate Medical School has shown that a quick daily rub with nettles over painful joints can bring relief to some who suffer from osteoarthritis. In this study the treatment reduced joint pain in nearly everyone and they reported that they preferred using nettles to their normal pain relief. What is more, 63 per cent planned to carry on using them. The prickling pain lasts for about thirty minutes, followed by a warm tingling sensation for up to twenty-four hours. This is perhaps the commonest cause célèbre instancing a herb under the microscope finally catching up with historical indications, anecdotal evidence and hundreds of thousands of cases that have benefited from traditional and folkloric medicine.

Upon skin contact, some individuals may get urticaria (nettle rash, hives). The root may also have some mild side-effects, such as gastrointestinal irritation, excess fluid production, or decreased urine flow. It may also alter the menstrual flow and, taken internally, enhance the effect of diclofenac, a non-steroidal anti-inflammatory drug. Do not take if pregnant, or while nursing.

DEVIL'S CLAW
Harpagophytum procumbens
SOUTHERN AFRICA

Devil's claw can be found growing wild in the desert areas of northern Angola and Zambia, in eastern Rhodesia, in the south of South Africa and in western Namibia. For thousands of years, various southern African peoples have used a decoction of this vicious-looking herb's tuber to treat digestive problems and arthritis. However, it was not until after the First World War that G. H. Mehnert, a settler in what is now Namibia, first drew the attention of pharmacologists to the remarkable results achieved with the herb by local people. Since then, it has been an effective therapy for rheumatism and disorders of the locomotive system. It is also used as a pain-reliever by arthritic and rheumatic sufferers worldwide.

In 1999 a German research paper called for devil's claw's use in the supportive treatment of rheumatism, and the plant was shown to improve motility and reduce pain in several clinical studies. Its active compounds are thought to be its glycosides, including harpagoside; this, or the related compound harpagide, is changed inside the body into harpagogenin, which may be the active ingredient that decreases the inflammation associated with arthritis.

Recently *Harpagophytum* was on trial again, this time in the treatment of knee and hip osteoarthritis. After a four-month double-blind trial it was found that the plant was at least as effective as the slow-acting osteoarthritis drug diacherhein, and that it reduced the need for analgesics and non-steroidal anti-inflammatory therapy. What a triumph for the afflicted, and for herbal medicine, and all thanks to an ancient and humble semi-desert plant from Africa.

BLACKBERRY
Rubus fruticosus spp.

Although fossil evidence shows that these aggressive plants have provided food for the human diet since very early times, black-berries remained a wildcrafted food until the nineteenth century, and modern families still like to go 'blackberrying'. The plant's use as a gargle to soothe sore throats was first recorded by the Greek physician Dioscorides during the first century AD. Called 'goutberries' in Europe well into the eighteenth century, they were also used by the ancient Greeks to treat gout and by the Romans for sore throats and inflammation of the bowel. Blackberry leaves were used in European folk medicine for wash-ing and staunching wounds, and traditional medicine also employs the roots and root bark for the same purpose; the fruits are used internally at both ends of the alimentary tract, to relieve inflammation of the gums, mouth ulcers and sore throats and as a remedy for diarrhoea, dysentery, haemorrhoids and cystitis.

Among its many health-giving constituents, the blackberry contains selenium, potassium, magnesium and pectin. There is anecdotal evidence building up in the United States that pectin, an old home remedy for relieving arthritis and rheumatism, does appear to help with pain relief (there, a branded product called Purple Pectin for Pain is on the market). There is also evidence to suggest that the whole fruit has much to offer those suffering from rheumatism and arthritis: recent research has proved that blackberries and their juice are antioxidant, their free-radical-scavenging power being at its height on the point of ripeness rather than when the fruits are over-ripe. So on with the black-berry vinegar, the blackberry desserts, jams and jellies of autumn, and lashings of blackberry syrup over the ice-cream at the end of a hard day's brambling in the countryside.

BLACKCURRANT
Ribes nigrum

EUROPE, ASIA, NORTH AMERICA

Blackcurrant is a fruit more associated with summer puddings than with medicine, and it is grown as a commercial fruit crop all over Europe. This is a good thing, since raw blackcurrants contain large amounts of potassium, calcium and phosphorus. They are also a great source of vitamin C and carotene, as well as antioxidant anthocyanin – all of these playing key roles in maintaining a healthy body. Blackcurrant has been used in the past to treat a variety of conditions, including diarrhoea and sore throats. It is now taken internally for problems such as adult eczema.

Recent medical research on the plant has focused on blackcurrant seed oil and the fatty acids it contains: blackcurrant seed oil is the richest source of omega-6 per weight of all vegetable oils. There is also some evidence that such essential fatty acids may enhance the effectiveness of calcium uptake, which may help prevent the development of osteoporosis. Other studies have shown that those taking blackcurrant seed oil experienced a significant improvement in morning stiffness and that it is a potentially effective treatment for active rheumatoid arthritis. It is now clear that blackcurrants and their oil provide a counterbalance to the inflammation that contributes to the deterioration of cartilage, resulting in damaged joints and bone surfaces and, finally, excruciating pain. The oil is now one of the components of a number of patented mixtures for the treatment of bone and joint inflammation.

BLUEBERRY
Vaccinium spp.

NEW WORLD

In America the diners' cry is 'Bring on the blueberry pie!' There are more than thirty-three types of blueberry to be found on that continent, where its health benefits have become widely appreciated. Now grown commercially in the USA, Australia and New Zealand, blueberries have traditionally been semi-managed by Native Americans, who would torch the scrub on acid lands, thereby allowing the blueberry bushes to proliferate – a practice that continues to this day.

At one time considered to be a useful diuretic and expectorant for catarrh and coughs, the plant has also been used to treat chronic skin conditions and even nervous exhaustion. Modern research is proving that it does indeed have a legion of sound medicinal uses. In particular, there is good news for sufferers of arthritis and rheumatism. It has been found that one of the fruit's most prized active agents, its flavonoids, and specifically its anthocyanosides, can stabilise collagen, the most abundant protein in the body and a constituent of veins, tendons, ligaments and cartilage. When joints, connective tissues, bones or cartilage are inflamed, collagen is destroyed, and it has been found that blueberry flavonoids help to prevent such collagen destruction and actually strengthen connective tissues. The anthocyanosides also inhibit free-radical damage and improve the tone of the entire vascular system by strengthening all the veins and arteries.

GREEN-LIPPED MUSSEL
Perna canaliculus

PACIFIC

Over a hundred years ago it was noted that eating green-lipped mussels, an amazing source of some of the body's most important chemicals, seemed to protect Maoris in New Zealand from developing arthritis. This marine mollusc has now become an accepted part of alternative medicine.

Green-lipped mussel extract contains all nine classes of glucosamines that occur naturally in the human body and are the building-blocks of the connective tissues. It can therefore help repair any of our connective tissues, including skin and joints. Glucosamines also help with joint compression and lubrication and can alleviate arthritis and suppress inflammation. The mussel extract inhibits the inflammatory effects of prostaglandin synthesis. This anti-inflammatory action has been found to be more potent than that of commonly prescribed pain-killers. Studies clearly show that extracts of green-lipped mussel can be effective in controlling painful arthritic conditions. The extracts are kind to the stomach, and so are beneficial when taken with non-steroidal drugs that are known to create stomach problems. Rich in vitamin B_{12} and super oxide dismutase, the mussel's nutrients also help maintain healthy blood cells and provide extra antioxidant protection for the body.

COMFREY
Symphytum officinale
EUROPE

Comfrey has been used for centuries to help heal wounds and mend broken bones. The plant native to wider Europe, from the Mediterranean to the Caucasus in the East and the British Isles in the West. It now grows worldwide wherever temperature and damp growing conditions allow. Another common English name for the plant is Knitbone. Comfrey gets its Greek name from symphyo, which means 'unite' and in Latin its name symphytum means 'to heal'. As this suggests, the herb's ability to promote the healing of broken bones, sprains and fractures has been known for thousands of years. A Greek physician of the 1st century AD prescribed it to heal wounds and mend broken bones. Later, Nicholas Culpepper in his 1653 'The English Physitian Enlarged ' recommended it in the extreme for broken bones, for sore breasts and haemorrhoids. In the past comfrey poultices were applied to external wounds and sores and a comfrey compress was considered very efficacious for a sprained ankle. Comfrey ointment continues to be used in proprietary ointments for bruises and sprains.

Research has shown that the root and fresh young leaves of comfrey contain allantoin which is well known for its ability to promote healing as a cell-proliferant that helps repair damaged tissue. The herb has always displayed anti-inflammatory action, which research indicates is in part due to the rosmarinic acid and other phenolic acids that comfrey contains. Comfrey infusions, tinctures and ointments for external use are considered safe, but current advice warns against self- medication. In accordance with the MCA and FDA and a voluntary agreement between MAFF and herbal manufacturers, no comfrey root tablets are made at this time. It is to be hoped that further investigation into the remedial properties of Comfrey will be forthcoming.

ROSEMARY
Rosmarinus officinalis
MEDITERRANEAN

Rosemary grows wild in the countries of the Mediterranean basin and in Portugal. Symbolic of fidelity and remembrance, it has become a well known 'pot herb' worldwide. It is one of those wonderful plants that fill the air with their perfume, and it is a herb not only for the body but for the mind and spirit too. It was burned for fragrance in the homes of the ancient Greeks and is still used by students when studying or before exams to help concentrate their minds. As well as being of importance in traditional Arab and Unani medicine, rosemary is now used in Chinese, European and Indian medicine as well as as a dietary supplement in the USA. It is used as a tonic, a stimulant and a carminative, and to treat digestive ailments such as dyspepsia. Rosemary oil is applied externally to alleviate poor circulation, or as a lotion for aching muscles and rheumatism. Rosemary-leaf tea contains useful amounts of phenolic antioxidants, and is effective against bloating, flatulence, nervous tension and mild cramp-like gastrointestinal and biliary upsets.

Research has proved rosemary to be a stimulant and a mild analgesic, whose properties are most easily applied via its essential oil. It has also been proved that the herb's oil has anti-inflammatory effects, chiefly due to rosmarinic acid and a flavonoid content, making it useful to those suffering from rheumatic and arthritic complaints.

Until 1926, rosemary oil was used in water to cleanse hospitals in France. There is perhaps a lesson to be learned from this quaint practice in the management of modern-day hospitals: in Britain alone there is an annual death toll of five thousand from infections picked up while in hospital 'care'. Even if today's professionals don't want to use this herbal disinfectant, perhaps a course of therapy using the essential oil might concentrate their minds on the immense remedial task ahead.

Rosemary oil may not be used in pregnancy or by epileptics.

11

Blood

Your blood consists of three main things: liquid plasma, 90 per cent of which is water, living cells called 'corpuscles' and cell bits called 'platelets' (already often mentioned in this book). Dissolved in the plasma are lots of proteins, albumin (the white stuff in chickens' eggs), globulins (some of which are very important to your immune system) and minerals, especially sodium and potassium. Platelets are continuously produced in your bone marrow, and there are on average an incredible 250,000 in every microlitre of blood. Small they may be, but they carry around with them very important chemicals that help the blood to clot and keep the walls of your blood vessels in good repair.

One drop of your blood should contain about five million living red cells (corpuscles) and five thousand white cells (also called 'corpuscles'). The red ones, unlike any of the other cells in your body, do not have a central control body, or nucleus, and so they do not live very long. Their job is to carry oxygen from the lungs to every part of your body where and whenever it's needed. They do this thanks to haemoglobin, a strange but very useful antioxidant protein that has a very useful and novel role in life. It contains iron, the same stuff the body shell of most motor-cars is made of. When exposed to water and oxygen the iron in that body shell combines with the oxygen to form red-brown rust. Inside our bodies much the same happens: the iron in our haemoglobin takes up the oxygen, producing oxidised haemoglobin, which is red. The haemoglobin then keeps this highly corrosive element, the iron, under control until it is safely delivered to those parts of the body where it is needed. Then and only then is it released ready for use.

Blood flowing in your arteries is full of oxygen and so is red, while blood flowing in your veins contains very little oxygen, so it looks blue. We go a bit blue when we get very cold, because in an attempt to conserve heat our bodies shut off the supply of blood to the skin. The blood trapped in the little capillary loops on the surface soon loses all its oxygen, and you feel as blue as you look.

Blue-baby syndrome, as its name suggests, is a condition in which the baby's haemoglobin is no longer able to latch on to the oxygen; the baby turns blue and can die. One cause is too much nitrate in its diet; this is a common component of all food and drinking-water, and a natural mineral usually in short supply but now becoming more abundant thanks to its excessive use in intensive agriculture. Nitrate has no such effect in adults, but in infants below the age of one the gut is less acid, ideal for digesting maltose but also ideal for the growth of bacteria that change nitrate into nitrite. Then the latter combines with haemoglobin to form metahaemoglobin – a substance that can't carry oxygen. Furthermore, there is now some evidence that high nitrate levels may increase the likelihood of stomach cancer. It is a sad reflection of the changing state of our environment that more and more people are choosing to drink bottled water. In many countries bottled water is now supplied to households with young babies.

The total length of blood vessels in an adult body is about 25,000 kilometres, the vast majority of them being tiny capillaries only 0.009 millimetres wide – just one-tenth the thickness of one of your hairs. As the red blood corpuscles are 0.007mm in diameter, that gives a clearance of only 0.001mm on either side, a fantastic feat of bio-engineering. With a traffic flow of 80,000 million cars – sorry, corpuscles – every minute, night and day, your internal raceway is enough to make even the most civil engineer a little envious.

Each red corpuscle lives for only fifteen days, after which it is scheduled for breakdown and recycling in your spleen and liver. Toxic waste is got rid of via your kidneys and iron is dumped with your faeces, giving them their rusty colour.

Over a lifetime of seventy-five years your heart will pump 268 million litres of blood around your body. That's more than 150 times as much water as you will ever use, despite living in a water-guzzling industrialised society.

Back to the cornflakes packet: cereals provide you with lots of fibre, which helps with bowel movements, plus a daily dose of iron to replace what you flush down the pan. Both are of great importance, for although *The Guinness Book of Records* doesn't include constipation, it can be a killer; so can anaemia, and every day your body must make 250 million new red corpuscles. These are being continually manufactured in the marrow of bones such as your ribs and sternum, and those production lines need a continuous supply of iron. In the bad old days before nutritional scientists had taught Mr Kellogg how to put the right sort of iron into his product, liver was the cure for anaemia – that is not having enough red blood cells in circulation. The patient had to eat it raw, and raw liver tastes horrible. Anaemia comes in a number of forms, all of which are treatable, if not curable. In this instance, it's *not* being in the red that makes you feel blue, so at the first signs, go and see the doctor.

Meanwhile, back inside your 25,000-kilometre raceway, your white blood corpuscles, a mere five thousand in each drop of blood, are doing a great job – you hope. Their task is to seek out and destroy – in fact, gobble up – harmful bacteria and unwanted bric-a-brac that get into your bloodstream. Each white cell is a mobile slaughterhouse and knacker's yard that engulfs and deals with all unwanted matter, thanks to the packets of digestive enzymes it contains.

These hard-working cells store information from all past attacks by disease-producing aliens and manufacture special chemicals called antibodies, which provide us with further and often long-term protection from infection. They then release the antibodies into the bloodstream, and if another attack takes place you may be certain that your guardian angels will recognise the foes by the antigen – the foreign substance – they carry. The white corpuscles will rapidly multiply, swelling the ranks of the defenders, and put the antibodies exactly where they will be most effective. Like all chemical warfare, this not only uses up a lot of your energy but also produces toxic waste – no wonder you feel proper poorly. When the enzymes and other systems expire, the corpuscles themselves are scheduled for destruction, so again, new ones have to be produced. And so on, all the time. Now you really know the meaning of a busy body.

These guardian angel white corpuscles are called 'leucocytes'. Leukaemia, characterised by too few white blood cells, is the result of one of the most dreaded forms of cancer. In recent times much research has centred on a family of plants that includes the blue periwinkles grown in our gardens. Their active principles are chemicals called vincristine and vinblastine, which are now helping in at least four out of every five cases of childhood leukaemia. But do not be tempted to experiment yourself – like many of our most promising herbal medicines, they are very poisonous plants.

The blood system is in effect a closed system. When intact and working properly, nothing can be squirted in at one end or out at the other. However, every day some three litres of water – that's more than half the total volume of your blood – is lost by diffusion through the walls of the capillaries. This water has to be replenished, and that's where your lymphatic system comes in. It's an open circulatory system in which open-ended lymph capillaries gather up body fluids by diffusion, passing them to ever larger ducts and on to two vein-like lymphatic vessels. These transport the fluids to the veins of the blood system through one-way valves. Similar valves positioned throughout the system direct the fluids along, pumped not by another heart but by the gentle squeezing of your musculature. It is thanks to your lymphatic system that the balance of water in your blood system is maintained. And it's a system that is so well hidden that we don't know we've got it until something goes wrong. Then all sorts of lumps and bumps appear as the lymph nodes swell up.

Achieving the first rung on the ladder to healthy blood has a lot to do with the calibre of the food you eat, which in the postmodern world has become 'the weakest link'. Everyone may want to become a millionaire and live to a ripe old age, but they are unlikely to be able to enjoy it unless they are feeling well – the best foundation on which to build happiness. In this twenty-first-century world home cooking and washing up may be awful chores, but a pizza with a squirt of garlic concentrate on it is about as far from the real thing as it can be. Also, when did you last get fresh parsley sauce on your fish and chips? And what about all that monosodium glutamate and added salt? No wonder high blood pressure and all those other so-called lifestyle syndromes are now beginning to take an ever greater toll.

PARSLEY
Petroselinum crispum
EUROPE, MEDITERRANEAN

Parsley was known to the ancient Egyptians, and was used by the ancient Greeks to crown their athletes and for ornamentation in funeral rites. In Britain, a thirteenth-century cookbook advised using parsley sprigs to decorate and add flavour to a variety of 'meates both boyled and roasted'. But today, with the demise of the traditional 'fish on Friday' routine and the accompanying parsley sauce, parsley is thought of as little more than a garnish, mostly to be seen wilting dismally on the side of the plate and left there uneaten. This is a great pity because mineral-rich parsley (which is a diuretic), along with liquorice and citrus fruits, is a natural blood-thinner that may help prevent clots. A rich source of calcium, iron, riboflavin, potassium, thiamine and other vitamins and minerals, parsley also contains a large amount of iron-rich chlorophyll – the darker the better.

APPLE
Malus sieversii
CENTRAL ASIA

The apple, which is today the commonest fruit grown across the world, is the stuff of myths and legends. From the ancient Greeks to the early Celts wandering from east to west with their Druid priests, many early peoples used the apple tree to nourish the spirit as well as to heal the body. It was the discovery of the technique of grafting by the ancient Greeks that led to the development of many clones, each with their own tastes, textures and fruiting times. From its roots to the tips of its branches, the apple tree shows just how versatile medicinal plants and herbs can be. The apple has been used for its medicinal value as a food, as a pulp poultice and as juice. Its uses have included battling against anaemia and hepatic insufficiency, and against demineralisation.

Science now tells us that apples are filled with powerful therapeutic agents: sugars, amino acids, vitamins, mineral salts, malic and tartaric acids and pectin. Studies show that eating apples daily over a three-month period can lower blood cholesterol, especially the 'bad' LDL type, by as much as 10 per cent. Rich in soluble fibre, which aids the regulation of blood sugar, apples help prevent a sudden increase or drop in the blood's sugar levels. This helps to reduce the risk of heart disease and is great news for diabetics. Pectin is also considered to play an important part in warding off heart disease, and although it may be taken in powder form, the fresh apple pectin produces better results. Apple juice aids the absorption of iron. Both the nutritional and beneficial digestive elements of the apple and its ability to detoxify the system furnish the fruit with the means to help fortify and 'cleanse the blood'.

Recent dental research advises rinsing the mouth with water and allowing forty-five minutes before brushing the teeth after eating an apple to avoid any damage to tooth enamel via lingering fruit acids and sugar. Other contemporary research makes plain that the apple's phenolics, procyanidins and other flavonoids indicate useful antioxidant protection for asthmatics and against the development of cancers. The apple's antioxidant benefits may even extend to cider. Long-term storage does not influence the fruit's flavonoid concentration or antioxidant capability. So even in this age of modern science, the old adage 'An apple a day keeps the doctor at bay' still seems to have a lot going for it.

PINEAPPLE
Ananas sativus

NEW WORLD

A native of South America, the pineapple is cultivated throughout the tropics for its fruit. This has been used traditionally to treat a variety of conditions and was believed to help relieve catarrh, arthritis, bronchitis and indigestion. Pineapple juice gargle has been used for sore throats. However, there's a great deal more to eating this exotic fruit than its cooling and soothing action against wind and gastric acid. The sour unripe fruit improves digestion, increases appetite and relieves dyspepsia. Pineapple has significant levels of pro-vitamin A, carotene and potassium, and is anti-inflammatory.

The reason for its anti-inflammatory disposition is not yet fully understood. One theory suggests that the enzyme bromelain that it contains blocks the prostaglandins that are a partial cause of swelling. Bromelain is a protein-splitter, easing digestion, and so it is a boon to those with protein-digestive problems. It hastens the repair of injured tissue resulting from general surgery, accident and diabetic ulcers, and has been used with some success to treat osteo- and rheumatoid arthritis. As the enzyme also reduces blood-clotting it may help remove plaque from arterial walls. One study suggests that bromelain may improve circulation in those with narrowed arteries, such as angina subjects, thus helping to relieve heart disease. Normally the fruit and juice are without hazard, but fresh pineapple can trigger allergic reactions in rare instances in sensitive individuals.

BURDOCK
Arctium lappa
EUROPE, ASIA

The latter half of that herbal double-act and favourite fizzy drink, 'dandelion and burdock', is known as the king of the blood purifiers. In North America, through the nineteenth and into the twentieth century, Burdock Blood Bitters was a famous patent medicine sold in the marketplace; now, only its empty bottles and other memorabilia may be found, as collectors' items for sale on the Internet. Native to Eurasia, burdock is grown in China, Europe and the United States and is a popular folk medicine around the world. Early Chinese physicians, as well as Ayurvedic healers, used it as a remedy for colds, flu, throat infections and pneumonia. Today, burdock seeds are crushed to make a favourite tincture to purify the blood. The volatile oils of burdock seed are

said to be diaphorectic, being used to induce sweating to help neutralise and eliminate toxins from the body. This aspect of the herb
is widely employed to support the kidneys in filtering acids from
the blood stream. Its alkalising action cleanses the urinary tract of
excess waste and uric acid. As a blood cleanser, burdock neutralis-
es most poisons and soothes the lymphatic system.

The protective effects of burdock on the liver are borne out by
research and are attributed to its rich armoury of antioxidants. It
also helps to restore gall-bladder function and stimulates the
immune system. Burdock contains vitamins A, B_1, B_6, B_{12} and
E, plus selenium. It has a high mineral content and studies show
that it is a good source of iron, as well as of the carbohydrate
inulin. Its chromium content helps regulate blood-sugar levels.
Burdock is considered a very safe herb and food product.
However, as with all herbs, when it is not home-grown the reputation and reliability of the supplier must be taken into account.

BEETROOT
Beta vulgaris var. rubra
SOUTHERN EUROPE

Beetroot was known as a vegetable as early as 300 BC. It was used
in ancient Greek and Roman cookery and was one of the foods
that the Greeks considered worthy of offering to Apollo at
Delphi. Today, the value of its roots is again being appreciated as
both a food and a medicine. The blood-purifying 'vitality plant's'
juice is often recommended for pregnant women and vegetarians
as an excellent source of folic acid and iron to combat anaemia —
shades of the Doctrine of Signatures, expounded by the Swiss
physician Paracelsus in the sixteenth century. Beetroot's high
folate content, plus useful amounts of iron, make it advantageous
to the liver, where venous blood containing digested food is
processed and which is the seat of vitamin A synthesis. Beetroot
is a good general tonic and an excellent liver, kidney and gall-
bladder cleanser. It also stimulates the immune system with the
purple-red antioxidants (anthocyanins and carotenes) it contains.

Recent research in the Slovak Republic has found that red beet causes a 30 and 40 per cent reduction, respectively, of serum cholesterol and triacylglycerol levels in rats. Don't forget that the fresh leaves are particularly rich in manganese. If beetroot juice doesn't grab you in winter, then that alpha-dish, Russian borscht, will do the trick, but be aware that beetroot contains a large amount of sugar (up to 8 per cent). Another passing fact well worth a mention is that, when used as a medicinal supplement, the red dye in beetroot, used commercially as 'beetroot red' (betanin), may colour faeces and urine red and pink, respectively. This effect, called 'beeturia', is harmless and disappears as soon as you stop taking the root.

RED SAGE 'DAN SHEN'
Salvia miltiorrhiza

CHINA

Salvias are evergreen shrubs and sub-shrubs of world-wide distribution growing mostly in the warmer temperate regions, favouring dry, sunny hillsides, little wonder that its name comes from the Latin *salvere* 'to be well'. Its purple-red roots gives it its English name and probably its association with blood. The herb has been venerated for thousands of years in China where it is employed both as a blood stimulant and as a safe effective remedy for many circulatory problems. The earliest of all Chinese herbal texts states that it 'invigorates the blood'. In Chinese medicine, Dan shen was used traditionally to treat conditions termed blood stagnation, or stasis, by decongesting coronary blood flow, assisting amenorrhoea (absence of menstruation), relieving dysmenorrhoea (painful and difficult menstruation) and obstructive uterine fibroids. Dan shen may also be inhaled and is even been incorporated into some Chinese cigarettes. In recent time science has become very interested in Red Sage and has confirmed the validity of the herb's traditional uses. Among its strengths, it is an excellent preventative for heart attack. 'Experimental studies have shown that Dan shen contains a compound tanshinone that dilates coronary arteries, increases blood flow, and scavenges free radicals in ischemic diseases, reducing the cellular damage and improving heart functions. Clinical trials also indicate that Dan shen is an effective medicine for angina, heart attack and stroke.' It is able to reduce angina symptoms and is more effective in treating chronic stable angina than the drug Sordi and provides support and preventive treatment for the heart's performance. Recent research reveals that a synthetic derivative of danshinone 'S-3-1' from Dan shen, a well known anticarcinogenic, might be developed as a new chemopreventive drug. Also intramuscular injections of S. miltiorrhiza have shown benefit in improving visual acuity and peripheral vision in people with glaucoma. Furthermore, the herb also contains a compound that significantly reduces cerebral infarction, which may be caused for example by the obstruction of a blood clot, prevents thrombosis formation and reduces neurological defects.

There is however evidence that Dan shen has a strong interaction with the drug Warfarin and can gravely interfere with anticoagulation control.

12

A Lot of Guts

There are nine metres of it, to be inexact, stretching from your mouth to your anus, which means that since the average adult torso measures about 75 centimetres all round as the stethoscope travels, your gut has to be coiled up. To simplify the matter, look upon yourself as what you are, a tube with attachments, or, in this twentieth-century world of fast food, a doughnut – elongated and convoluted for convenience, maybe, but that is what you are. That hunk of gorgeous you is able to live it up thanks to a hole down the middle.

The hole down your middle is your alimentary canal, or gut, and food glorious food goes in at the top and what's left of it plops out at your bottom. While the food is in your gut it is in effect still outside your body, or at least outside the main works, and you should thank your lucky stars that it is because in its undigested state it would be poisonous. Yes, if you took your favourite four-course meal, liquidised it and injected it into your bloodstream, you would probably die, for all that stuff must be processed and made compatible before it gets inside your body.

Plants are made of plant proteins and people of people proteins. If the proteins that go in at the top went straight into your bloodstream they would immediately be recognised as foreign bodies by the antigens they carry and be dealt with by your white corpuscles. Before they pass from outside your main organs to the inside, they must be broken down into their component amino acids, which don't carry any antigens and so don't trigger your immune system. Your body then accepts them for use as building-blocks for your own unique proteins, which are plastered with your very own antigens. This is why for skin grafts and organ transplants identical twins make the best donors. The rest of us are so unique that our body parts will be rejected unless stringent precautions are taken.

The process by which our food is made acceptable by our internal system is called digestion, as we all know, and to make it happen the lining of the 'hole' is very complex and is connected to a number of other complex organs: three pairs of salivary glands, a pancreas and a very large liver all well supplied with blood vessels and nerves. It would in fact be true to say that the concentrated plexus of nerve cells associated with your digestive system is your second brain.

No wonder, then, that as early as 1857 it was realised that those problems of digestion, especially ulcers, are inextricably linked to mental activity, and anxiety in particular. Peptic ulcers are caused by the fact that to aid the digestion of meat and all the other proteins and to kill off unwanted bacteria, our stomachs produce lots, and I mean lots, of hydrochloric acid. Nasty stuff – tankers carting it around our roads have to carry warning notices. The problem is that our guts are also made of protein, so if anything goes wrong with the protective lining of your stomach or the bit immediately below, it gets the acid-bath treatment. You begin to digest yourself from the outside in, opening the tissue up to attack by bacteria, and this results in a gastric or duodenal ulcer. Our modern lifestyles simply ooze anxiety.

No wonder, in view of all this, that food dictates so much of our behaviour from the moment we are cut off from our prenatal lifeline, the umbilicus that connected us to our mums. From that moment on, our gut reaction shapes our every day. The ritual of eating has bound the family together from the gathering around the fire at the mouth of the cave to the 'Don't get down until you have finished' command that used to keep us in touch around the table – one more reason why fast food has not done much for family life.

When I was young, Sunday lunch, which often included a salad, started with grace, and Dad would say, 'Lettuce pray.' This is the first joke I can remember. Like all vegetables, lettuce is pretty indigestible for the simple reason that plant cells are made of cellulose, the same stuff that makes up the bulk of tree trunks and paper. Not surprising, therefore, that much of it is going to go right through, as part of that all-important roughage that helps our food on its way.

PREPARATION

All foods need to be broken down to aid digestion – that's what molars are for. And the more you chew, the more satisfaction you gain, for your tongue and your nose allow you to savour the taste and aroma. It always amuses me to see wine buffs savour the vintage with great care and then swill it down as they bolt their food. Mastication is a do-it-yourself way of heightening the pleasure of eating and of ensuring better digestion. Chewing not only reduces the food to smaller and smaller bits, increasing the surface area on which the digestive juices can get to work; it also warns the stomach that food is on the way, so gets the juices flowing.

The first juices to be added are from the salivary glands, and though these glands are relatively small they do produce a lot of saliva. Surprise yourself: chew a piece of gum and instead of swallowing your saliva, spit it into a glass and see how much you produce in, say, ten minutes. You could have a competition to find the family champion. Whether you win or not, your saliva contains a range of your very own food additives: enzymes, whose sole function is to help smash up proteins, fats and carbohydrates, the very stuff of which you are made. The saliva immediately gets cracking on the giant starch molecules, beginning to break them down into their component sugars ready for you to use.

Oral hygiene shouldn't stop when you grow up. Indeed, if only we had always brushed every morning, before bed and after meals, those toothaches, visits to the dentist – and, dare I say? dentures – might never have happened. The only good thing I have ever heard about the latter is that if anything goes wrong with them you simply hand them over to get them fixed. There is now good evidence that dental cavities are caused in the main by our intake of refined sugar – two spoonfuls, please – in the form of sweets, cakes, biscuits and so on. In the old days we used to take in more starch, as opposed to today's predominant sugar, so that the enzymes released the sugars lower down, well below tooth level. As far as my teeth were concerned I was a lucky wartime baby, for both sugar and sweets were on ration.

The trouble is that bacteria thrive on sugar, and they don't have any teeth to worry about. Gums awash with sugar from that nightcap, however innocent, breed bacteria by the billion, plastering your teeth with plaque and boring holes into the bargain. Always use your tooth-brush before you go to bed, then perhaps you won't ever have to wake up in the morning with your dentures in a glass beside the bed. And you will also be a nicer person to wake up with. A tooth cavity can con-tain millions of unwanted bacteria, all living it up at your expense. They don't even try to get out for a pee, so all their waste collects in the cavity – no wonder your breath smells bad in the morning. It has been estimated by the World Health Organisation that one dentist to every thousand people is necessary to keep our teeth healthy. That means that the world ought to have six million dentists.

Fortunately, many millions of people in what we should call 'the smiling countries' have less need of the dentist's high-speed drill. They still have a real national health system in place – it's called a wholefood diet. There is, however, one problem faced by all the teeth in the world: they can be damaged and contract infections that eventually kill them. A dead tooth can then become a seat of infection and lead to granu-lomas and abscesses. The most dangerous tooth infections are those that cause no toothache, remain undetected but become a silent source of toxins which, when carried around the body, lead to all sorts of other disorders. So regular visits to your dentist are a very sensible notion, for an X-ray can reveal hidden facts that could mean life or death to you or (preferably) to those bacteria. (Remember, too, when sitting in the dentist's chair that he or she may be just as worried as you are, for when it comes to stress, research has shown theirs to be among the top three professions.)

In the days of long sea voyages in sailing-ships, once the supplies of fresh vegetables and fruit had run out, the long-suffering crews developed that terrible disease called scurvy. Their breath stank, their gums rotted and their teeth fell out. The cure was ready and waiting in every port: a little bright-green plant growing on the shore that they called 'scurvy grass' (see p.204), and they called it that for a reason – it helped cure the problem just described. Only later did they discover that it was rich in ascorbic acid, or vitamin C. Thank goodness that today we get fresh vegetables and citrus fruits even in the middle of our annual cruises through winter.

The arguments both for and against the fluoridation of drinking-water will rage until we stop drinking the stuff. The 'fors' point out that they add it only at the rate of one part per million and that in some drinking-water it is naturally present in much higher concentrations. The 'againsts' state that over their lifetime people are being forced to drink much more fluoride than would ever be necessary to keep their teeth in good repair, and that fluoride in large amounts is a deadly poison.

Dental floss is made of the lint from the fruits of the cotton plant, first grown in India. Today it is an important part of oral hygiene, especially in those countries whose children crave fast food. The twigs of the neem tree (see p. 224) have long been used in village India as toothbrushes; its bark contains a bitter substance, refreshing the mouth with no need for peppermint, and the wood fibres are tough but not abrasive. As all winegum addicts will know, there is nothing better than a real hard chew to get the blood flowing through the gums. It carries the toxins away and speeds fresh supplies of oxygen and nutrients, including calcium and fluorine, to rebuild the protective enamel.

At the back of your teeth your body's strongest muscle, your tongue, is firmly anchored. Not only does it allow you to taste sweet, salt, bitter and sour, it helps to break down your food and knead it into a ball and enables you to enunciate the words that communicate pleasure or disgust. Behind your tongue, your epiglottis has the crucially important job of closing off the top of your windpipe every time you swallow. If it didn't, the food could fall down into your lungs, choking you to death. As long as the epiglottis does its job, the food, well lubricated with saliva, passes on towards the stomach.

Oh, I almost forgot your tonsils and adenoids. Tonsillitis, though mainly a childhood affliction, can strike at any time. The old 'pull 'em out at any sign of trouble' cure has given way to the 'leave them be' syndrome of the age of antibiotics. Tonsils and adenoids, in their healthy state, are small masses of lymphatic tissue, and as such are part of your main line of defence against infectious organisms attacking your ears, nose and throat. They are therefore best left where they are.

STAGE TWO

Meanwhile, you have swallowed, and the food is in your oesophagus on its way to the stomach. It is helped along your gut, whose walls are made up of layers of special smooth muscle that never tires, by peristalsis. This is a process in which regular waves of relaxation, followed by waves of contraction, gently push the food on its way. Your stomach is then ready and waiting to produce two main enzymes, pepsin and rennin, plus lots of hydrochloric acid, which allows the enzymes to get to work. Pepsin helps smash up big proteins and rennin does the same to the proteins in milk.

It may not taste very nice, but raw carrot, cabbage and especially potato juice prepared fresh in the juicer are nature's own Alka-Seltzer. Squeamish? Then try blueberry juice or chew a stick of liquorice – much more effective than after-dinner mints to calm the stomach and the mind. When I was young I used to chew woody liquorice roots with relish. Well, the bright-yellow juice is sweeter by far than sugar, and instead of causing harm it can settle your stomach. Those suffering from peptic ulcers should say a big thank you to the carbenoxolone produced by the light-blue flowers and seedpods of the liquorice plant, for it was the greenprint for the highly effective synthetic carbenoxolone, which helped make ulcer surgery almost obsolete.

THE REST OF THE JOURNEY

The gentle churning in your stomach slowly but surely reduces the food to a soupy consistency, the stuff you throw up from time to time. Vomiting is perhaps the most spectacular way in which your body tries to get rid of poisons like caffeine and alcohol. The latter is the only substance that passes directly into your bloodstream from your stomach – that's why you get drunk so quickly and, if you continue imbibing, your stomach reacts in self-defence. Nasty acid taste, isn't it? Vomiting aside, only when the time is right does the stomach open up the valve at the bottom, letting regulated squirts of part-digested food through into your duodenum until the stomach is empty. The acid chyme, which is what the stuff your stomach produces is called, must be neutralised very quickly, or duodenal ulcers could add to the problems of indigestion, for the enzymes of the rest of your intestines only work in an alkaline environment.

As soon as the acid hits the top of the duodenum it sends out messages via the blood to the pancreas, telling it to start releasing a whole portfolio of enzymes. These include trypsin, which chops up the proteins into amino acids, and into a consistency fine enough to pass through the wall of the intestine into the blood. The enzyme amylase now attacks the big carbohydrates, and lipase snips away at those long-chain fats. The digestion of fats is aided by the emulsifying agent, bile, which is produced by the liver and collects in your gall-bladder ready for use. Gallstones are hard concretions made of cholesterol, plus calcium and a yellow pigment made by the liver. Ten per cent of the American population and 20 per cent of all those over fifty have them. Collecting in the gall-bladder or the bile passages, they can cause a painful condition called cholelithiasis, the fifth most common cause of hospitalisation among adults.

The lining of the small intestine is covered with millions of fingerlike projections called 'villi'. These are in constant motion, waving about and expanding and contracting. They are well supplied with blood vessels and extensions of the lymphatic system called 'lacteals'.

The food has by now been processed by digestion into small building-blocks: amino acids, simple sugars and fatty acids. The first two move into the blood, dissolve in the serum and are pumped around by the heart to every part of the body. The fatty acids move more slowly through the lymphatic system squeezed along by the surrounding tissues until they re-enter the bloodstream via a vein near the heart. What's left of the food – the indigestible bits and sufficient roughage, you hope, to give peristalsis something to work against – is now in a very fluid state, thanks in the main to the water added with all those enzymes along the way. Water is very precious, so one of the main functions of the large intestine is the resorption of water and the formation of solid faeces. Not too liquid and not too solid, but just right for plopping out – a neat package of organic manure.

Most of us have at one time or another suffered the inconvenience of diarrhoea. Something goes wrong, bacteria get out of hand, a population explosion of baddies takes place, poisons accumulate, water is moved in to dilute them, giant gas bubbles form. The pain is excruciating, for the smooth muscles find themselves out of kilter doing unusually hard work. Charcoal in the form of tablets or biscuits is a great stopper-upper, and taken after one of the hard-hitting drugs that effectively deal with acute diarrhoea (even Montezuma's revenge), it certainly helps to restore normality. One thing always to bear in mind is that these superdrugs often clobber the goodies along with the culprits. So natural unpasturised yoghurt is a good way of restocking your gut with the bacterial flora it and you require. If you happen to be in the tropics where amoebic dysentery may be the cause, don't hang about but go straight to the doctor.

Chronic but less spectacular forms of diarrhoea are best treated with a change of diet and lifestyle. Less worry, less raw fruit and vegetables, no cooked cabbage, or anything that causes flatulence. A short period of fasting, to give the whole system a well earned rest, won't do any harm. Bananas are mild constipators, and along with apples and potatoes (especially when baked in their jackets) can do a lot to help.

Two valves, or sphincters, close the lower end of your bowel: the first you can't control, and it opens under pressure to let the faecal masses through into the chamber below. Normally you have full control over the lower anal sphincter, but when you have to go, you have to go. Most of us go once a day as regular as clockwork, while some people only need to go every two or three days.

It has been estimated that at least one in every five American adults is constipated, and half of them are regular users of laxatives. Poor health, a poor diet and nervous tension cause constipation. The main problem is that the longer the waste products stay in the bowel the more water is resorbed, so they become drier and harder to pass. Also, with legions of faecal bacteria feeding on them, more gas is produced; and more unwanted waste, theirs and yours, plus poisonous chemicals may pass through the wall of the lower gut into the bloodstream. Constipation is your own internal doctor warning that something is wrong and that something is allowing poisons into your system. Laxatives only relieve the symptoms and are not in themselves a cure. But do have a care, as the cause of constipation might just be a malignant growth getting large enough to obstruct the motion. Likewise, untreated constipation could trigger such a growth. It has been said that 'death lies in the bowels', and today it's a fact that cancer of the colon fills more and more operating rooms; and more and more mortuaries prove the point.

In recent times, almost half the patients referred by their GP to a gastroenterologist (a gut specialist) are found to be suffering from irritable bowel syndrome (IBS), a condition which affects up to one third of the UK population. The symptoms are abdominal pains, constipation often alternating with diarrhoea, flatulence, anorexia, anxiety or depression. The causes are many, the latter two symptoms being high on the list of suspects. Excess production of gas can put pressure on the spleen, causing pain in the lower chest and left shoulder, increasing both the spasms of the intestine wall and the worry factor. Extensive tests may rule out organic causes for symptoms such as these and point, rather, to the portfolio of lifestyle syndromes that afflict twenty-first-century man and woman.

Two other bowel conditions, also very common in Western fast-food societies, are diverticula disease and haemorrhoids – the sags and the piles. And please remember that you can't entirely blame the fast food – think about the lifestyle that goes with it. Snacking is bad not only for Garfield the really fat cat, but for you as well; it never gives your guts a chance to rest, and if it's always soft processed food that you're snacking on it gives them little to push against. So the wall of your bowel starts to sag, forming pockets, or diverticula. These tend to trap the waste, especially that all-important roughage that should be being pushed along. Trapped too long, putrefaction can occur causing not only a nasty stink but also inflammation leading to a much worse complaint, haemorrhoids.

Piles result from weakened blood vessels in the wall of the anal canal, the last bit of your gut before the long drop, forming their own diverticula which are a sort of varicose veins, little grapelike bags of blue deoxygenated blood that can remain hidden or hang out the bottom. Either way, you know you've got 'em. The pain and the burning irritation are unbearable, and pushing against a hard, dry stool can make them burst.

Wholemeal bread, bran and brown rice are all good sources of dietary fibre and will keep you regular. However, don't go mad if you are not used to the stuff. This is especially important if you have diverticula disease, in which case agar products made from seaweeds will ease things along. Algae, or seaweeds, are almost a staple of the Japanese diet: they have nori with breakfast and nori or wakame at lunch and dinner. Remembering our marine origins and the health record of the Japanese, it can't be a bad thing. The mineral content of seaweeds is very similar to that of seawater. Seaweeds, as we have already seen, also contain a whole range of nutrients including vitamins A, B, C, D and E, amino acids, fats and enzymes, all of which they manufacture themselves under organic conditions. And it isn't just the Japanese who appreciate the virtues of seaweed: the Welsh used to start the day with laver bread, the Scots used to rave about dulse and the Irish, Irish moss (or carragheen). We modern Celts seem to have forgotten how good it tastes and how it can keep us on the highroad to health. The age-old use of seaweeds as fertiliser along the coasts of the Celtic fringe certainly showed that our ancestors understood the importance of trace elements, especially iodine, in which seaweeds abound.

If you *have* to snack, its great to nibble raw wakame (20–34 per cent protein, 1,400 milligrams of calcium and lots of iron in every 100 grams consumed); I share it with my cats, and they love it too. Unfortunately, it binds to itself heavy metals and radioactive substances when it gets the chance. (Wakame was used to rid survivors of Nagasaki of their radioactive load.) So be careful which beach you collect it from: not too close to Windscale – sorry, Sellafield – and check the origin on the packet.

As far as bowel movements are concerned it's the alginates, which give them that sticky but slippery feel, that are important. Though non-fibrous and with nothing to get trapped in the gut, alginates take up water, swell and add nice soft bulk, just like it should be. For all landlubbers strawberries, indeed any fruit that makes good jam, contain lots of non-fibrous roughage in the form of pectin. This is what stops the fruit from falling to pieces and makes real jam rather than the stuff now called 'preserves'. Pectin also swells with water, putting bulk in the way of peristalsis. So believe it or not, strawberries will help keep you on the move. Rhubarb, one of the prizes of the early trade routes to China, increases the flow of saliva, settles the stomach and though a purgative when used in large doses has long been used in the treatment of diarrhoea.

Recent research indicates that the incidence of cancer of the colon is three times higher in those who abuse alcohol and indulge in so called 'empty-calorie diets' than in those whose diets are rich in the folate vitamins and the amino acid methionine. On the other hand, moderate drinkers with well balanced diets rich in fresh fruit and vegetables do not have a greater risk of cancer.

PEPPERMINT
Mentha x piperita
EUROPE, ASIA

Mint leaf is seldom far from a real cook's mind, and it is also one of humanity's oldest herbs, for there is evidence of peppermint cultivation in ancient Egypt. In the history of the mints *M.* x *piperita* is a relatively new natural hybrid that first appeared in an English spearmint crop about three hundred years ago. The parent herbs are native to Europe, Japan and China and the hybrid is naturalised in North America. Refreshing peppermint is known for its invigorating qualities, and its essential oil contains menthol, menthone and menthyl acetate as major components. More than just an after-dinner mint, in the West the herb has been primarily employed for gastrointestinal upsets, both as a remedy and as a preventive. Russian herbalists use peppermint infusions to treat gall-bladder inflammation as well as flatulence. Following extensive research, the internal use of peppermint oil has been approved for, among other ailments, spastic discomfort of the upper gastrointestinal tract and bile ducts, and irritable colon.

A recent breakthrough has been the use of enteric-coated (kind to the stomach) oil-of-peppermint capsules for irritable bowel syndrome (see p. 194). Of hospital patients who took (Obbekjaer's) oil-of-peppermint capsules for four weeks, over two-thirds reported an alleviation of their symptoms. The antispasmodic activity of the oil is the major feature, relaxing the smooth muscles of the intestine and stomach. Peppermint's antiseptic and anaesthetic actions, as well as the anti-ulcerogenic effect of its flavonoids and its antioxidant properties, may also be helpful in easing the symptoms. The old uses for peppermint oil and leaf hold true, but this new discovery is likely to be of great assistance to many people. We often hear of placebos kidding the patient back to health. Now you know it, peppermint really works; go ahead and savour those After Eights. However, mints and mint tea are not a choice for the anaemic, as peppermint may interfere with iron absorption.

CARAWAY
Carum carvi

Caraway, a widespread flavoursome and aromatic herb, has been used since ancient times to calm the digestive tract and expel gas. Caraway seeds have been found in food remains from 3500 BC. The plant is mentioned in the Egyptian Ebers papyrus of c. 1500 BC, and the Greek Dioscorides advised caraway to aid digestion. In 1996 it was chosen as one of the new industrial crops sanctioned by the European Union to be grown for its essential oils. Western traditional herbal medicine employs it for appetite loss, fever, liver and gall-bladder problems, bronchitis, colds, cough, and other common infections. It has also been used to improve lactation and induce menstruation. It is a pungent herb, and in India is used medicinally as a carminative and stimulant, although it is perhaps better known today as a culinary spice. Universally employed as an antispasmodic and digestive, and for flatulent dyspepsia, it is a secondary herb for colic and gingivitis. Caraway has something of a reputation for easing heartburn. Its astringency is useful for treating diarrhoea and laryngitis (as a gargle).

In 1990, the D-limonene in caraway oil was among compounds found to inhibit the tobacco-specific carcinogen NNK, so it may have the capacity to diminish the carcinogenic response to exposure to tobacco.

Used as a tea in modern Egypt, caraway has been found to facilitate the absorption of iron in the intestines, and it also helps to prevent ulcers. Caraway oil in enteric-coated capsules, in conjunction with peppermint oil, has begun to be used as a treatment for irritable bowel syndrome. This combination was compared with the patent medicine cisapride and found to provide an effective and safe means of treating dyspepsia.

SLIPPERY ELM
Ulmus rubra

A wonderfully soothing preparation celebrated in Country and Western songs, the secret having been learned by the settlers from the locals, the bark of this aptly named tree is full of demulcents. After brushing your teeth, there's nothing like a good slippery-elm gargle to start or end the day. The herb is found mainly in the Appalachian Mountains and in Mexico and has been cultivated as a street tree in the USA. It is a tried and tested Aboriginal remedy and is used in Ayurvedic medicine as a primary nutritive tonic. Native Americans used it in many ways: as a healing salve (made from the outer bark), as a poultice for wounds and inflamed eyes, as a drawing remedy for boils and internally for ulcers.

As a herbal remedy, the mucilaginous, 'slippery' inner bark is excellent for digestive-tract problems, and is so good for the bowel that the most recent research (2002) suggests it should be formally evaluated for its efficacy in the treatment of inflammatory bowel disease. Although its use is restricted in some countries, slippery elm bark is an official drug in the United States and is used for dysentery and other bowel diseases, cystitis and irritation of the urinary tract, and as an enema. The herb is used internally to treat gastric and duodenal ulcers, colitis and infantile digestive problems. Because of its generous complement of vitamins, minerals and trace elements with antioxidant effects, all of which promote vitality and reinvigorate debilitated systems, slippery elm is employed as a food for the weak and convalescent, from infants to the elderly. In its powdered form it is also considered to be a kindly baby food. Slippery elm's curative actions are well understood and are based on its ability to soothe inflammation, to detoxify and to coat any irritated tissue with its protective mucilage on contact.

It should be noted that taking slippery elm with oral medications might decrease their absorption. So take it at least several hours before or after.

PSYLLIUM
Plantago ovata and other spp.
EUROPE, ASIA

Psyllium, a member of the plantain family which includes many common-or-garden weeds, has a long history of medical use as a safe and effective laxative. For thousands of years it has served well both conventional and traditional systems of medicine throughout Asia, Europe and North America in cases of constipation. It has a bulking action that is beneficial to diarrhoea, irritable bowel syndrome (IBS), ulcerative colitis and Crohn's disease. The seeds swell when moistened into a gelatinous mass, promoting peristalsis and hydrating the faeces, so easing the motions. And there is help for haemorrhoid sufferers too, in the herb's ability to soften the stools and reduce the irritation of the affected veins.

Research in the 1980s demonstrated that psyllium has both a laxative and an anti-diarrhoeal action, helping to restore normal bowel function. More recent studies have looked at its effect on chronic constipation in association with IBS, with good results, finding psyllium seeds to be more effective than wheat bran. To date there have been no reported ill effects for the domestic use of this herb, except for one case of allergic asthma in a 'constant care' setting that involved twice-daily use (which is more frequent than is usually called for).

MUNG BEAN
Phaseolus aureus
ASIA

The mung bean, or green gram, is a nutritious protein food plant that has been used for thousands of years. It is often eaten as sprouts, a live salad supplement that has become popular in the West since the 1960s. Gram for gram, mung bean sprouts have the carbohydrate content of a melon, the vitamin A of a lemon, the thiamine of an avocado, the riboflavin of an apple, the niacin of a banana and the ascorbic acid (vitamin C) of a loganberry. Mung beans also contain large amounts of fibre and protein, iron and folic acid. In Central America the leaves were used in baths to treat rheumatism and rickets. Oriental herbalists used the beans for all inflammatory conditions, ranging from systemic infections to heat stroke and hypertension. They are an antidote to toxic poisoning and have been shown to be very effective taken as a soup for heat stroke, alleviating thirst, irritability and fever.

It is thought that the sprouts have a regenerating effect at a cellular level because of their high concentration of RNA, DNA, protein and essential nutrients. The enzymes they provide are also very important for the body's life processes. Enzyme depletion is a fundamental cause of ageing, and as we grow older enzyme loss can make us more susceptible to disease. The sprouting process goes hand in hand with the generation of chlorophyll, which has been shown to be effective in overcoming protein-deficiency anaemia. Indeed, the rejuvenating and life-giving properties of mung bean sprouts may be one of the hidden health secrets now germinating across the world.

GENTIAN ROOT
Gentiana lutea
EUROPE, ASIA

Gentian root is obtained commercially from wild plants in the mountains of France, Spain and the Balkans. The plant is said to take its name from King Gentius of Illyria (reigned 180–167 BC), who, according to Pliny the Elder (c. 23–79 AD) and Dioscorides, was the first to discover *G. lutea*'s therapeutic properties.

In Europe, gentian and other intensely bitter plants have been used for centuries to settle the stomach, to aid weak digestion and to counter flatulence and poor appetite. Called *longdan* in Chinese, gentian is used for inflammatory conditions associated with problems such as jaundice, hepatitis and hypertension. It is used in Ayurvedic medicine for the circulatory and digestive systems as a bitter tonic and for its antipyretic, bactericidal and laxative properties. In cases where the system is debilitated by disease, too, gentian makes a good tonic, especially after exhausting fevers, and it has been used against malaria instead of quinine.

Gentian's reputation for stimulating digestive function, including the production of stomach acid, has been validated in modern times. Research has shown that the active principles are the bitter substances contained in the herb, which excite the taste receptors, leading to an increased secretion of saliva and digestive juices. When used as an appetiser and for indigestion, it is the iridoids in the gentian root and rhizome that are thought to be likely to stimulate gastric secretion in humans, as they have been shown to do in animals. Gentian is now the most popular of all gastric stimulants and widely used to treat all types of gastrointestinal disorders, including dyspepsia, gastritis, heartburn, nausea and diarrhoea. The extract reportedly aids the secretion of bile by the liver and stimulates a greater bile flow.

CLOVE
Syzygium aromaticum
ZANZIBAR

One of the earliest spices to be traded, cloves were imported into Alexandria as early as 176 AD and are said to have reached Europe c. 300 AD. Clove was first mentioned in Chinese medicine c. 600, and traditional Chinese physicians have long used the *din xiang* herb to treat indigestion, diarrhoea, hernia, ringworm and other infections. India's traditional Ayurvedic healers used *lavanga* to treat respiratory and digestive ailments. The flower buds, which are used in Western and most other medical disciplines, contain a volatile oil consisting chiefly of eugenol.

In modern Western herbalism, cloves are considered to be an aromatic antiseptic, a stimulant, a carminative, an anti-emetic and an anodyne. Their strongly antiseptic property makes them useful in many areas. Clove oil is used for toothache – it will stop pain when applied direct – and for oral hygiene. In common with many culinary spices, clove kills intestinal parasites and exhibits broad antimicrobial properties against fungi and bacteria, which is in line with its traditional use against diarrhoea, intestinal worms and other digestive complaints. It is good for digestive discomfort such as abdominal bloating, flatulence, dyspepsia and colicky pain. A few drops of oil in water will arrest vomiting, and clove tea, too, is used to relieve nausea.

Japanese researchers have discovered that, like many spices, clove contains antioxidants that help prevent cell damage. In research carried out in the UK in 2000, clove oil considerably inhibited the effects of twenty-five genera of bacteria, which included food-poisoning and -spoilage bacteria. In 2002 researchers have been contemplating the use of clove oil to prevent the formation of fungal toxins in grain destined for rural communities in South Africa.

ANISE
Pimpinella anisum
EUROPE AND AFRICA

Anise, or aniseed, is a member of the carrot family and originally came from Egypt, North Africa and Asia Minor. It was cultivated as a spice by the ancient Egyptians for at least four millennia and later by the Greeks, Romans, Chinese and Arabs. Aniseed is now grown worldwide. In his *A New Herball* (1551) William Turner wrote that 'anise relieves pain, but also sweetens the breath'. Other early English herbalists recommended the herb for many problems including hiccups, asthma and bronchitis. In Ayurvedic medicine it is considered a carminative and a stimulant, and thought to induce milk flow in lactating mothers. In China it is an anodyne, a carminative and a stimulant, and is used against cholera and kidney complaints. Elsewhere it is used for colic, to cool the stomach and for gonorrhoea. In the West, as an expectorant, it is a common component of cough mixtures and lozenges.

Anise seed is well known for its ability to reduce wind and

bloating and acts as a natural antacid to settle the digestion. Aniseed is used for its antispasmodic properties to alleviate period pain, asthma and whooping cough, and against respiratory ailments as an expectorant. It calms coughs, helps with bronchitis, improves memory and counteracts oily skin. Even today it is said to increase milk production.

The herb is rich in phytochemicals and contains many minerals and vitamins, in particular vitamin A. Its volatile oil (1–4 per cent), chiefly trans-anethole (70–90 per cent), provides the basis for its internal use to ease griping, intestinal colic and flatulence, as it helps prevent fermentation and gas in the stomach and bowels. It may also reduce the effects of morphine in mice, which could have some future use in drug-dependence treatments. The oil is narcotic and in large doses slows circulation.

SCURVY GRASS
Cochlearia officinalis

EUROPE

In the highlands of Scotland where it has traditionally been cultivated, this cause célèbre of a food medicine is called *am maraiche*, meaning 'the sailor', and has been a favourite food of seadogs from Viking times. John Gerard's great *Herball* of 1597 lists its main virtue as being a cure for scurvy. Sadly, it was not until 1795 that the British Navy bowed to herbal wisdom and included an ounce of lemon juice (a much more transportable source of vitamin C, which we now know does the trick) as a compulsory ration while at sea. Scurvy grass was taken at breakfast as late as the nineteenth century, and used as a poultice for boils or cramps. This wonderful weed also contains glucosilinates, a volatile oil, a bitter tannin and minerals. Mainly used as an antiscorbutic and diuretic, it has antiseptic and mild laxative actions. The juice is used as a gargle and mouthwash for ulcers and sores in the mouth, and topically for spots and other blemishes.

CORIANDER
Coriandrum sativum

Coriander, cultivated as a medicinal herb by the ancient Egyptians, Chinese, Indians and Greeks, was introduced into the British Isles by the Romans. Ayurvedic medicine employs the herb for cystitis and urinary-tract infections, for skin conditions such as urticaria and other rashes, and for allergies and hay fever as well as vomiting and indigestion. In Russia, coriander's effectiveness as a digestive herb is legendary, and it has been used as such for centuries.

Introduced into Chinese medicine and cooking c. 600 AD and named *hu*, meaning 'foreigner', it became the herb of immortality. Recent Japanese research suggests that it suppresses the accumulation of lead in the body. Chinese herbalists today use the seeds to treat indigestion, anorexia, stomach ache and influenza. Chinese folk medicine uses coriander leaves (Chinese parsley) and seeds to remove unpleasant odours from the genitals of men and women, as well as for halitosis and bad breath. In the West, apart from the traditional gastrointestinal use of this anti-fungal herb, aromatherapeutics employ coriander oil for muscular aches, poor circulation, neuralgic pain and nervous exhaustion. It is also effective against certain food poisonings.

In one of the world's oldest cookery books, *De Honesta Voluptate et Valetudine* ('On Right Pleasure and Good Health') written by the Italian physician Bartholomaeus Platina in 1480, the author makes clear the herb's importance and describes in painstaking detail how to concoct the perfect coriander and carrot sauce. More recently, tom yum gung soup, liberally laced with coriander, has been found to be an anti-cancer agent. Irish research has shown that coriander is a useful treatment for diabetes, while recent trials in India have found that it may be effective against colon cancer.

WILD STRAWBERRY
Fragaria vesca

Adults and children alike prize this mouth-watering fruit, especially the wild variety. The strawberry has become a culinary pleasure, with fruits eaten fresh, added to summer drinks, juiced for flavour or made into desserts. Seemingly little employed in the West until the Middle Ages, it has often been given scant attention as a healing herb. In 1652 Nicholas Culpeper reported that 'the berries are excellent good to cool the liver, the blood, the spleen or a hot cholerick stomach, the leaves and roots thereof also good to fasten loose teeth and to heal spongy foul gums'. More recently the leaves and roots have been used in teas and infusions in cases of diarrhoea and digestive upset, and the fruits are used externally for 'face masks' to counteract skin blemishes and sunburn. The juice can be used to remove stains from discoloured teeth. In Europe the fruit has been prescribed as part of the diet in cases of tuberculosis, as well as gout, arthritis and rheumatism. In Ayurvedic medicine, the mildly diuretic leaves are used as a 'cooling' astringent, helping to heal wounds. A grand jam-maker, the pectin in strawberries greatly aids the digestive system.

Nowadays, the strawberry plant can boast a far greater role than mere gourmet's delight, for we know that it contains all the minerals required for a healthy body except iodine and that it's a very good source of potassium. The sunshine fruits have much vital energy: carotene, and all the vitamins except A, D and B_{12}. All herbalists agree that the strawberry is efficacious in treating kidney-stones and joint pains and celebrate its overall tonic effect. Finnish research has proved it to be antimicrobial, antibacterial and antioxidant in the raw.

13

The Waterworks

Well, you hope the waterworks work. Constipation is bad enough, but the inability to pee when your bladder is full is excruciating and deadly. Normal bladder volume is around 750 millilitres (that's almost two pints) although it can hold a lot more. The pain is due to the fact that your bladder is made of smooth muscle which objects to being made to do too much work, and it signals the fact in a most effective way: Please pee, and let me off the hook. Your own cold feet on the bathroom floor or someone else's on your back in bed, a cold draught, fright, stress, strain or anxiety can also make you want to pee.

Your kidneys are two large bean-shaped organs that lie in the small of your back, one to each side, just outside your body cavity. Your guts fit in between, suspended in a shock-absorbing peritoneal fluid; but your kidneys don't have that advantage, so rugby-players beware! Each kidney consists of about a million highly sophisticated filtration and reabsorption units all well supplied with blood pumped through tiny capillaries. Water and poisonous wastes like urea, ammonium ions and creatinine are pressure-filtered from the blood into the mass of small capillaries, or glomerulus. Small as these are, they have been shown to receive 75–100 litres of effluent a day. Thank goodness most of the water content is secreted back into the body through the walls of the renal tubules before the rest is stored in your bladder. (If this were not the case you would have to keep drinking and peeing all day, or your bladder would be the size of a bath.) To achieve this, the living cells that make up the tubules have to do a lot of hard work.

Remember those hormones and your master gland, the pituitary, dangling down from your brain? Well, one of the chemical messengers it produces is called pitressin – and with a name like that it must have something to do with the water works. Pitressin tells the kidney tubules to keep the pumps hard in reverse, keeping the precious water in while concentrating the waste ready to be shipped out.

Sugar is another substance transported by the blood and under hormonal control – two hormones, to be exact: adrenaline, produced by the adrenals, and insulin from your pancreas. After a good meal there's more sugar circulating in your blood than the body can use. Insulin tells your body to store it away as glycogen, exactly where it will be needed in your muscles. Similarly, when the moment arrives adrenaline commands, 'Turn it back into sugar ready for action.' If this were not the case we would all have to keep exercising hard and eating all the time to keep sugar levels under control. Today diabetics can keep their insulin levels up to scratch by regular injection. Excess sugar in the blood is not the result of kidney trouble but of malfunction of the pancreas; in the old days diabetes was diagnosed by means of the physician tasting the urine for sweetness.

Malfunction of the kidneys is signalled by all sorts of things appearing in the urine, like proteins and sugar. With proteins, it's caused by an increase in blood pressure forcing them through the filter, while sugar indicates diabetes. Blood in the urine, on the other hand, may indicate kidney disease or damage. Never treat this as a flash in the pan, but go and see the doctor without delay. That is, unless you have been eating beetroot (see p.184), for there are certain harmless water-soluble pigments that just naturally pass on through.

One of the conditions that show up in the urine is 'type 2' or late-onset diabetes, which is on the increase. Called 'late-onset' because until recently diabetes was mainly confined to the over-forties, the disease is now appearing in children and teenagers across the world and seems to be related to obesity and a sedentary lifestyle. 'Type 1' diabetes is an auto-immune disease in which the body appears to destroy its own insulin-producing cells. In the United States, the incidence of type 2 diabetes rose from 4.9 per cent in 1990 to 6.5 per cent in 1998, in both sexes, across all ages, ethnic groups and education levels, and in nearly all states. *Diabetes now costs Britain's National Health Service nearly a tenth of its budget.*

Of course, the search is now on to find the genetic basis of this new epidemic, and two genes have been identified that may be related to it. Type 2 is less well funded and less well hyped than type 1, but there is now conclusive evidence that if risk factors associated with excess weight, lack of exercise and poor diet were addressed, this could substantially prevent the onset of the disease, delay its progression and even reverse some of the symptoms. A community-based project pioneered in Karelia by the Finns three decades ago, proving that lifestyle changes could help in the prevention of heart disease, broke new ground, to the extent that the Finnish Diabetes Prevention Study Group was inspired to carry out research designed to discover whether modifying diet and lifestyle could prevent type 2 diabetes developing in people at high risk from the disease. The study involved 522 middle-aged, overweight subjects aged forty to sixty-five, all of whom had impaired glucose tolerance – that is, after eating or drinking, glucose was slow to clear from their bloodstream.

The total incidence of diabetes after four years was 11 per cent in the group that was treated, compared to 23 per cent in the control group. During the trial, the risk of diabetes was reduced by 58 per cent in the first group: 63 per cent lower among men and 54 per cent lower among women. These results were highly significant. There were also other improvements in the treated group: decreases in waistline measurement, blood glucose and insulin both on fasting and two hours after eating, in blood triglycerides and in blood pressure. In other words, subjects in this group were generally healthier.

Results from the first three years of the Diabetes Prevention Program in the USA show that regular exercise and a modified diet have reduced the incidence of type 2 diabetes by 58 per cent among patients with impaired glucose tolerance. The study, conducted in twenty-seven medical centres and involving 3,234 people, found that diet and exercise were more effective than the drug metformin in preventing the disease. The trial ended a year early because the data had clearly answered the main research questions.

HOP

Humulus lupulus

EUROPE

The hop is a member of the plant family that includes cannabis and has had early associations with man through its use in the making of bitter beer. The therapeutic use of the plant in Europe

---

dates back to at least the ninth century, and hops have a long and proven history of herbal use, employed mainly for their soothing, sedative, tonic and calming effect on both body and mind. In Indian medicine hops are used for restlessness, and in traditional Chinese medicine to treat insomnia, dyspepsia, intestinal cramps and lack of appetite. A pillow stuffed with aromatic hop flowers has long been a popular means of procuring sleep, and today in both Germany and the United States hop infusions, tinctures and dry extracts are used in sedative preparations. It is now officially recognised that hops may be beneficial in cases of mood disturbance such as restlessness and anxiety, as well as sleep disturbances.

Modern research has found that the hop's bitter principles generally stimulate the digestive system and that two of these, lupulon and humulon, are antiseptic. The hops essential oils and extracts have been shown to have antibacterial activity and some of its constituents are sedative, while others have chemopreventive properties. Hops are one of the richest sources of phyto-oestrogens, and recent research suggests that these might be used in dietary supplements to treat menopausal symptoms. Beer is rich in anti-cancer properties, and people who drink it in moderate amounts may reduce the risk of heart attack, heart disease, strokes, gallstones and kidney-stones – and a daily Guinness comes highly recommended during pregnancy and the menopause.

DANDELION
Taraxacum officinale
EUROPE, ASIA

You all remember the story about dandelions and wetting the bed? Well, it's true if you eat them, for they contain a diuretic that can help the urine flow smoothly. And the white sticky stuff that oozes out of the broken leaves and stems helped the Russian army to move smoothly during the last world war. Cut off from supplies of tropical rubber, they used the next-best thing. Raising thousands of hectares of this weed, they used its latex to make tyres for their war machines. But 'weed' is perhaps a word we should use with great care now that we are beginning to learn that plants have all the answers.

The wonderful dandelion is a bit of a gypsy. Originating in Europe, it has parachuted into temperate zones all around the world. A member of the daisy family, its name initially derives from the Arabic *tarakhshaqun*, 'wild chicory', and its leaves were recommended in the works of Arab physicians in the eleventh century. The herb has been a regular food medicine, and once sustained the inhabitants of the island of Menorca through a famine. It contains high levels of potassium salts and its store of vitamin A (beta-carotene) is higher than that found in carrots. It also contains vitamins C, B complex and D, mineral calcium and one and a half times more iron than spinach. Dandelion is a well known liver and kidney aid; it also cuts the fat and helps eliminate or drastically reduce acid indigestion and gas build-up. It is the herb's leaves that are used chiefly as a diuretic and tonic, and it has been said that they are a potential equivalent to frusemide, a drug obtained on prescription for treating hypertension. Recent research on mice has suggested that dandelion extract may act against diabetes – a promising result.

Dandelion is generally considered safe, even in large quantities and for unlimited duration. However, those allergic to the daisy family may get a contact reaction or may develop mouth sores. Those with bile problems should consult a healthcare practitioner before eating dandelion. It should also be avoided if you are taking lithium, as its diuretic properties may lower sodium levels and cause the lithium to increase to a toxic level. Dandelion may also interact with other diuretics, lowering the effects of those medications.

CRANBERRY
Vaccinium macrocarpon
NEW WORLD

A food medicine to the North American native peoples, cranberries first appeared on the modern dinner table as a sauce to accompany the festive turkey, adding its antiscorbutic marvels to the diet of the early European settlers. Cranberry is today one of those summer fruits we take for granted. Its juice is a key remedy for the alleviation of recurrent cystitis and to prevent further problems in this department. It is also suggested that it may be an immunity booster and useful to the elderly for urinary-tract infections. So 'Clean out the plumbing with cranberry!' should be one of the calls for a healthy lifestyle.

While its efficacy is proven, not everyone agrees on why cranberry juice keeps problem bacteria at bay. According to researchers at the Alliance City Hospital, Ohio, in 1985, as well as containing large amounts of vitamin C, gallic acid and anthocyanosides, all natural antibiotics, cranberry juice seems to have a 'Teflon effect', stopping bacteria from clinging to the inner walls of the urinary tract and so allowing them to be flushed out in the urine. Up to 60 per cent of women will experience at some stage the discomfort of urinary-tract infections (UTIs), and some will recur. In 2002 a Finnish study showed that highly antioxidant cranberries can alleviate *E. coli*-induced UTIs by up to 85 per cent, while cranberry and cloud berry juice concentrate may reduce UTIs by about half.

Cranberries are antiviral and antifungal, but alas they have no effect on the *Candida albicans* fungus that causes thrush. For those suffering from kidney-stones, *small* amounts of the fruits may be useful to help lower the level of calcium in the urine, thus aiding the prevention of stone formation. However, cranberries are quite high in oxalates, which can encourage kidney-stones, so it is wise not to eat too many or drink too much of the acidic juice, and it should not be given to infants. Remember, as with all raw fruits, to wash the berries to avoid any environmental contaminants.

CHICORY
Cichorium intybus
EUROPE, MEDITERRANEAN, ASIA

Chicory belongs to the same family as the dandelion, endive, salsify and sconzonera – all vegetables worthy of culinary and herbal attention. A bright-blue-flowered wayfaring plant, it occurs in temperate zones and in western Asia and North Africa, and is now extensively cultivated. Both wild and cultivated chicory was known to the Egyptians and mentioned by Horace, Ovid, Virgil and Pliny the Elder, and according to the latter it was good for headaches and, when mixed with wine, for efficient liver and bladder function. Today, as in the sixteenth century, the roasted, ground root is sold mixed with coffee or as a coffee substitute, and chicory leaves (blanched by forcing shoot growth in the dark) are found prepacked in plastic bags in the supermarket. Medicinally chicory acts as a diuretic, tonic and laxative. Like dandelion, it is said to have a cleansing action on the urinary tract. In Ayurvedic medicine it is also used as an alternative, a diuretic and fever fighter.

Experiments have shown that the components lactucin and lactucopicrin, which contribute to chicory's bitter taste, may counteract the effects of caffeine by their sedative action on the central nervous system. In 1998 inulin, one of chicory's main components, was considered in the *Annual Review of Nutrition* for its potential use as a risk-reducing agent for a wide range of diseases including non-insulin-dependent diabetes. As with many other herbs, yesteryear's predictions for chicory may become tomorrow's science! Indeed, the latest research suggests that chicory's inulin may protect against colon cancer, and that *fructooligosaccharide* (FOS), which can also be isolated from chicory root, may increase the helpful bacteria in the colon as well as increasing calcium absorption and faecal weight, thereby shortening the transit time in the gut. With the added promise of decreasing the amount of lipids in the blood, inulin tablets are already being sold in Finland.

JUNIPER
Juniperus communis
EUROPE

Juniper, which gives gin its distinctive flavour, should be all right for the gin-and-tonic set. It also contains an active diuretic – no wonder they make so many trips to the little boys' room. And the tonic, with no lack of human guinea-pigs, is still doing Trojan work as an anti-malarial. Furthermore, recent research using animals has shown that in conjunction with other traditional herbs, in a Croatian formula called 'Antidiabetis', juniper is hypoglycaemic and may have a useful contribution to make to the management of type 2 diabetes.

Herbal treatment should not last longer than four to six weeks. The oil should not be used by those with inflamed kidney disease, although the herb is OK. Do not use oil or herb extract to make home-made cosmetics or toiletries. Neither the oil nor the herb should be used in pregnancy because it is an abortifacient, as recently proved in animal experiments.

BUKO, YOUNG COCONUT MILK
Cocos nucifera
PACIFIC

In the Philippines and elsewhere, coconut provides many things for the indigenous populations: oil, beverages, cream (*gata*), vinegar (*suka*, from the coco palm), a jam (*matamis na buo*), a syrup (*macapuno*), an after-dinner sweetmeat (*bukayo*), an alcoholic drink (*tuba, lambanog*) and a vegetable. Its husk is used as a floor polisher (*bunot*), as a building material and for firewood, and charcoal made from the shell gets hot enough for firing pottery. The husk is now exported as coir, a substitute for peat in the horticultural industry, and used in many other products around the world.

But one of the plant's greatest wonders is what they call in the Philippines 'nature in a chalice', coconut water (or milk) drunk straight from the nut through a straw. It is called *buko*, which means 'young coconut milk'. This refreshing diuretic drink sold on the street recently became especially popular with the young, who used it in combination with 'Perla soap' for dealing with sexually transmitted diseases (STDs), although *buko*'s supposed efficacy in this respect was considered myth and hearsay by the establishment.

In the 1980s Dr Eugenio Macalalag, chief urologist of the Philippine army's general hospital, attempted to restore this traditional medicine to favour by putting one aspect of its use, the prevention and removal of urinary stones, to the test. He called the process 'bukolysis', and his extensive researches showed that oral buko therapy, using fresh *buko* water, *buko* nectar concentrate or *buko* nectar concentrate powder, dissolved all kinds of kidneystones. He also found that some of his patients were able to suspend dialysis treatment after regularly consuming this coconut water.

In 1996, when it was doing a roaring trade out on the streets, *buko* suffered a setback: samples were found to contain a poison. Despite the fact that the alien substance in this newly manufactured product was shown to be formalin (presumably added to increase shelf life), demands were made to remove *buko* from the marketplace. It is to be hoped that more open-minded research will be done on it in the future, and that another 'gift of nature' cure is not allowed to fall into the abyss of professional jealousy.

14

Take a Big Breath

The quintessence of a healthy life is a breath of fresh air, and so it should be because oxygen kills bacteria. Poor little things, you might think, these simple cells totally lacking in internal membranes, many of which evolved before their photosynthesing relatives poisoned their environment with oxygen. One of the strangest facts of life is that oxygen, once free inside a cell's protective overcoat, will kill it – and that includes our cells too.

The seat of this conundrum lies in the fact that proteins are made of chains of amino acids that depend on a simple sulphydryl group (a sulphur atom joined to a hydrogen atom) to keep them in shape and in working order. If oxygen gets to them, it steals the hydrogen from the sulphur, which immediately links up with other sulphur groups to form molecular bridges, screwing up the proteins so that they can no longer work. Likewise with all those internal membranes made of polyunsaturates and the fat-soluble vitamins A and E: oxygen does them no good at all.

Luckily, haemoglobin, the pigment that makes our red blood cells red, comes to the rescue. Haemoglobin traps the oxygen and holds it safe out of harm's way until the heart delivers it to exactly where it is needed. If any oxygen escapes from this high-security transport system, there are those special self-sacrificing chemicals that we have encountered already in this book: antioxidants, which mop up any spare oxygen. Important among these are vitamins C and E which, like the polyunsaturates that make up so much of our important working parts, cannot be manufactured by our bodies; they have to be obtained from our food.

Before we understood all this, some premature babies placed in oxygen tents went blind: their optic nerves oxidised away before their mothers had provided them with the antioxidants they needed. Inside your mum, of course, your lungs contain no air at all – all the oxygen you require is supplied via the placenta. A slap on the back from the midwife and the first breath changes all that; from that moment on you have left your aquatic habitat behind and your lungs contain just enough air to keep them partly inflated. At each breath the average adult inhales only about half a litre and exhales the same amount: this is called your 'tidal air'. An extra big breath can take in another three litres, the 'complemental air', and a real effort at breathing out will expel a litre, your 'reserve air'. Even then there's another litre and a half of residual air left inside.

Add tidal, complemental and reserve together and that really gives you something to boast about – your own VC (your vital capacity). This is the amount of air you can shift in flat-out exercise. Although you are born with a certain basic potential in this department as in others, training can certainly improve your VC and give you a chance of going for gold.

Your trachea, the bit closed off by the epiglottis when you swallow, leads down to your bronchi, which branch out into bronchioles and finally into small blind sacs called 'alveoli'. The walls of these are well supplied with capillaries through which blood is flowing all the time. It is here that the vital exchange of gases takes place between your blood and the outside world.

Each new breath of tidal air is rich in oxygen and poor in carbon dioxide compared to the reserve air, which is about half a metre away in the alveoli. Likewise, the air in the alveoli is richer in oxygen and poorer in carbon dioxide than the blood in the capillaries. So in an attempt to bring it all into balance oxygen moves in and carbon dioxide moves out by the natural process of diffusion, aided by your mass transport system, breathing.

At rest, we move about seven litres of air a minute, producing in our noses a wind speed of 2 on the Beaufort Scale. In flat-out exercise we shift 100 litres a minute (a wind speed of 7 on the Beaufort Scale, signifying a 'moderate gale'). The more work you make your body do, the more oxygen you use up, the more carbon dioxide is produced and the faster your lungs have to work. The lungs are made to work by the muscles of the chest and diaphragm, not by expanding and contracting themselves. Elastic bags they may be, but they are suspended in a closed chamber, your thorax, which is surrounded by fluid. To make you breathe, your muscles simply increase the volume of your chest cavity, thereby reducing the pressure inside the lungs and making fresh air move in to restore the balance. One trouble is that as the diaphragm moves down it may find a beer belly in the way. Excess fat puts a strain on everything.

The other thing that tends to get in the way of breathing is a bunged-up nose, and living in a temperate urban environment where the common cold is common indeed and flu is far from uncommon; one often wonders why we have a nose at all. But noses are in fact useful things, performing three vital functions: as a heat exchanger, a humidifier and an efficient filter. Bony structures called 'turbinates' whirl the air around the nasal passages. These are lined with living cells that are well supplied with tiny hair-like cilia, which wave about as well as secreting mucus, and so are both warm and wet.

The hairs and the mucus trap microscopic particles – pollen grains, dust, soot and the like – in the incoming air, preventing them from reaching the more delicate exchange membranes down below. The cilia all work in unison, doing their best to move the mucous mass back towards the nostrils where a handkerchief is hopefully waiting. Coughs and sneezes do spread diseases perhaps more effectively than we think, for calculations indicate that a short sharp cough generates nasal winds in excess of the speed of sound. Your nose should therefore be classed as a supersonic weapon of germ warfare. (Mine, unfortunately, was downgraded by the London Irish Rugby Club.)

Noses are immensely important, and you should always breathe through them – this is even more important these days when our lifestyles fill the air with all sorts of pollutants. First we had the smog, a lethal mixture of soot and sulphur dioxide. Our noses did their best with the soot, and our snot bore witness by turning black. The sulphur dioxide, being a gas, went right in and got to work on the lining of the inner recesses of the lung, causing pulmonary oedema. Sounds nasty – well, it is, for it means that body fluid is oozing into the lungs where it can be lethal. To prove it, a weekend of smog in London in 1952 caused at least four thousand extra deaths, speeding up government action to ban the inefficient burning of cheap, sulphurous coal. Up went the price of heating, and the venting of sulphur dioxide shifted to the taller chimneys of electricity-generating stations, which dumped the stuff far and wide, resulting in the dreaded acid rain. Some thirty years on and at immense cost, we got around to fitting power stations with 'scrubbers' (apparatus for removing impurities).

Meanwhile, in both urban and rural environments, the internal combustion engine reigns supreme: spewing out acidifying oxides of nitrogen, carbon monoxide (a killer), low-level ozone (a carcinogen), particulate carbon and rubber eroded off your speeding tyres – all part of a fricassée of transboundary pollution, which means it gets up everyone's noses. The carbon pours out of even well tuned lorries, especially when they are negotiating our crowded towns; have you ever bothered to ask, 'Why are they here?' The towns can't cope with them, so why should we? With billions of particles all about the same size as bacteria, our nasal mucosae just cannot cope with the onslaught. No wonder the incidence of respiratory problems is soaring: in winter it's sore throats, sinusitis, bronchitis and pneumonia; in summer, hay fever and asthma are on a massive increase.

Here are some of nature's own warnings – please take note:

* *sore throat* Your body's warning that something is wrong. Barley (*Hordeum* spp.) water and barley sugar have long been favourites for soothing sore throats (in use since the time of the pharaohs).
* *strep throat* An acute infection of the throat caused by bacteria called streptococci.
* *bronchitis* An inflammation of the bronchial tubes producing that deep, throaty cough, which is the body's way of trying to clear up the problem. Be warned: 75 per cent of all cases of chronic (long-term) bronchitis are smokers.
* *pneumonia* Inflammation of the inner membranes of the lungs, especially those of the alveoli, which often follows on if the above conditions aren't dealt with. Bacteria and viruses can cause pneumonia (viruses are the cause of more than 75 per cent of all acute pulmonary infections). Note: antibiotics do not kill viruses.
* *sinusitis* An inflammation of the mucous membranes, which swell up, blocking the tubes and making it difficult for even supersonic sneezes to clear the way.
* *hay fever* An allergic reaction causing the dilation of local blood vessels and the swelling of nasal and respiratory mucosae, clogging the whole thing up.
* *asthma* A condition affecting twice as many boys as girls under

the age of ten. Allergic reactions can cause constriction of the bronchioles, so holding the stale air in and leading to suffocation, spasms and even death.

The last two are certainly triggered by specific chemicals in, especially, pollen, fur and feathers to which certain people are allergic. This always was part of the rich tapestry of life, nature's own background of organic chemicals, a sort of seasonal homoeopathy that our bodies tuned into or succombed to. Such allergy is now on the increase, and part of the cause is pouring out of all those exhaust pipes. Children used to walk to school exercising their legs and lungs in pure air, rich in pollen grains at certain times of the year. Now they ride in state, exposed to whiplash and pollution from other people's exhalations, the latter recirculating within the confines of the family car.

In the same way, the elderly, many of whom can't afford to run a car, are forced to breathe the stuff as they try to make their way around towns and cities designed for cars and not for people. No wonder the incidence of all respiratory complaints is going up. With more and more of those body fluids oozing into our lungs, allergies are on the rampage. There used to be a sign outside a township in America that read: 'Last year twenty people in this town died of gas. Two inhaled it, two ignited it and sixteen stepped on it.' On a nationwide scale those figures are sure beginning to skew in the direction of inhalation.

Hiccups and pleurisy are not afflictions of the airways and lungs, respectively, but of the parts that make them work. While on the subject of airways and, come to that, air-conditioning, all that ultra-dry air we breathe in does our lungs no good at all. Warm, damp air is what our noses like getting stuck into, and a humidifier in the bedroom can work wonders. Back to hiccups: hiccups are caused by stimulation of the nerve that runs across your diaphragm. Again, it's water to the rescue! Drink it cold from the far side of the glass – it may dribble down your front but it will stop the hiccups.

Pleurisy is an infection of the membranes that line the pleural cavity, and a life-threatening condition if not properly treated. Early in the last century, before antibiotics, pleurisy-root (*Asclepias tuberosa*) was the most popular cure. Now it has been found to contain a specific substance that inhibits the growth of certain bacteria, including those that cause tuberculosis. Research is going on apace, especially as certain forms of the once dreaded tubercular bacteria are now showing resistance to antibiotics.

THYME

Thymus vulgaris

EUROPE, MEDITERRANEAN

Thyme is one of those common herbs that can be counted among the aristocrats of medicine. A native to the Mediterranean basin and vast in variety, thyme grows wild in many places in Europe and North America and is cultivated all over the world. An unidentified species grew in ancient Egypt, and remains of *saem* (T. spicata) were found in the tomb of Tutankhamun. Thyme may also have been used in the embalming process, and it still grows in Egypt today. It was known to Hippocrates, Dioscorides and Pliny the Elder, and it still fills the air with its perfume on the slopes of the Hymettos hills in Greece, renowned for their healthful thyme honey, which is frequently used as a respiratory-infection medicament. Little wonder, then, that HRH Prince Charles chose the plant for his celebrated Thyme Walk at Highgrove, where the lightest tread will be rewarded by an uplifting scent from under foot.

Nicholas Culpeper (1616–54) described the herb as 'a noble strengthener of the lungs, as notable a one as grows, neither is there scarce a better remedy growing for that disease in children which they commonly call the Chin-cough [whooping cough]. It purgeth the body of phlegm and is an excellent remedy for shortness of breath.' Indeed, thyme was traditionally used mainly as an antiseptic against infections, especially respiratory ailments such as bronchitis and pleurisy in adults and whooping cough and asthma in children.

Now in Britain, thyme or garden thyme (*T. vulgaris*) is used as a carminative, a tonic, an antiseptic, an antussive, an expectorant and a spasmolytic. The versatile herb contains volatile oils, especially thymol, as well as flavonoids, caffeic acids and tannins. Its myriad compounds can be taken internally or inhaled. It's thought that thyme's high antioxidant content partially explains why the tough men of the Caucasus mountains, who include wild thyme in their daily diet yet smoke, drink and make merry, enjoy good health with impunity. In Russia thyme is used as an analgesic, an antimicrobial, an astringent, an antispasmodic, a carminative, an expectorant and a tonic. An extract of thyme is part of Pertusin, an official medicine in the former Soviet Union for bronchitis and whooping cough.

Do not use thyme in pregnancy. And although it contains many immuno-boosting antioxidant phenols and flavonoids do not use it in excess, as there is limited data on its interactions with other nutrients and drugs.

ICELAND MOSS
Cetraria islandica
EUROPE, ASIA

Iceland moss is in fact a lichen that flourishes on heaths and hilly crags, and has recently come to the fore as a respiratory remedy. However, in northern Europe it has long been used in bread, and when gelled can be mixed with lemon, sugar, chocolate or almonds to make confections. The yellow-green lichen is employed in Scandinavia and Europe to stimulate the appetite and relieve dry coughs and inflamed tissues of the mouth.

Recent research has given a nod of official approval to the traditional use of Iceland moss in lozenges for the prevention and treatment of sore throats: 'It provides an advisable therapeutic opportunity without interactions and side-effects for the treatment of inflammation of oral mucosae occurring after nasal surgery.' Research has also shown that Iceland moss is antioxidant and immunologically active. Its lichen acids are effective against organisms such as salmonella, which causes gastrointestinal ailments in man and beast such as food poisoning, gastroenteritis and septicaemia. The plant also contains about 60 per cent important water-soluble and hence digestible polysaccharides, the basis of its use as a famine food.

Stop-press news and further food for thought: the University of Illinois has found in this common lichen compounds that inhibit an enzyme essential to the replication of HIV. AZT and three other AIDS drugs that have been approved by the FDA do the same thing, but it's been shown that these drugs are toxic and do not completely inhibit the virus. The lichen constituents, on the other hand, were found in laboratory studies to be non-toxic to cells, which would indicate that it is a safe food medicine (and, I have no doubt, a very useful addition to soups and salads).

HORSERADISH
Armoracia rusticana
EUROPE, ASIA

Horseradish is a 'blow yer head off' traditional condiment for the Sunday roast and a homely herb producing conspicuous head-clearing effects, as well as now a mainstay of sophisticated sushi bars. The pungent plant was known to the Egyptians in 1500 BC and grown in Greece more than three thousand years ago. Legend has it that the oracle at Delphi told Apollo: 'The radish is worth its weight in lead, the beet its weight in silver, the horseradish its weight in gold.' A biblical bitter herb of the Jewish Passover, it was in medieval times regarded as an aphrodisiac, used in a folkloric cough syrup and regarded as a cure-all.

During the Renaissance the consumption of horseradish spread to Central and Western Europe; by the sixteenth century it was used in cordials and in England became *the* accompaniment to beef and oysters. Calling it Raphanus rusticanus, John Gerard said in 1633: 'Horse radish stamped with a little vinegar thereto, is commonly used among the Germans for sauce to eate fish with, and such like meates as we doe mustard, but this kind of sauce doth heat the stomach better, and causeth better digestion than mustard.' The English took it to the New World, where in 1844 Henry J. Heinz, having helped his father grind and jar the herb in the basement of their home, produced horseradish as one of the first condiments of the modern age.

Apart from stimulating the digestion and increasing gastric secretions and appetite, horseradish has a long reputation for being effective against infection of the urinary tract (supported today by the use of horseradish root in the American urinary antiseptic drug Rasapen). Its capacity to facilitate perspiration has long made it useful for feverish colds and flu. A rich source of vitamins B_1, B_2 and B_6, it is mainly used alleviate bronchitis, the common cold, sore throats and sinus congestion. It is now known to contain a volatile oil, isothiocyanates, and glycosides with antibiotic properties. In laboratory tests it has killed the human influenza virus, and has done the same in vivo in animals. Its ability to alleviate throat and upper-respiratory-tract infections is widely accepted. All good enough for the German Commission of Herbal Medicine to approve the use of horseradish both internally and externally against catarrh, as a supportive therapy for infections of the urinary tract and as a treatment for minor muscle aches of the sort that usually bedevil the body when you have a cold.

So if you've got a lot on your plate, need to clear your head, warm your stomach or kill off cold infections go off to the sushi bar. However, never use too much horseradish, and keep it away from your eyes. Do not use if you have hypothyroid problems or stomach ulcers, intestinal or kidney disorders. Avoid using it during pregnancy or while lactating, and never give it to infants.

NEEM

Azadirachta indica

INDIA, SRI LANKA

Neem is known as 'the village pharmacy' in India, where it has been used for at least four thousand years in folk and then Ayurvedic medicine, and it still provides some of the most widely used herbal remedies. Neem is a 'holy tree'; traditionally its leaves were strewn on the floor at weddings and used to cover the body at death. Neem twigs make an efficient toothbrush with a built-in antiseptic paste, and the leaves are an effective natural insecticide.

Mahatma Gandhi was a regular drinker of neem tea and sang the praises of its wealth of nutrients and healing properties. Bronchitis has long been treated with a combination of oral doses of neem leaf tea twice a day along with inhalation of the steam produced by boiling the leaves. The steam contains volatile oils and aromatic compounds that, when inhaled and backed up by the oral doses, reduce the inflammation and attack the disease agents directly. In experiments with cattle, when neem oil is included in the feed the number of lung infections is significantly decreased when compared to the control group.

Neem has been found to be antiseptic, bactericidal and antiviral, and to strengthen the body's overall immune responses. Research has found that neem contains meliacins, triterpenoid bitters, tannins and flavonoids, plus a substance called 'nimbidin' that can reduce the spasmatic effect of nicotine by up to 90 per cent. Neem also has a calming action on the nervous system, which may reduce the desire for nicotine and the anxiety associated with it. Neem extract might, then, offer a means of reducing the effects of nicotine while enabling smokers to stifle the addiction.

WATERCRESS
Nasturtium officinale
EUROPE, TEMPERATE ASIA

Watercress is native to Europe and temperate Asia and is naturalised and cultivated in North and South America and the West Indies. It is found growing wild in wetlands in the UK and elsewhere, particularly in areas with hard calcareous water. It is a long-established tonic food, and Hippocrates (c. 460–377 BC) was probably the first physician to use watercress for its expectorant action. In India, the powdered leaf has long been used as an expectorant in the treatment of bronchitis. Valued since ancient times as an antiscorbutic, it has always been noted in times of war as a reliable source of blood nutrients. Watercress is a purifying herb; Culpeper in the seventeenth century used its juice as a lotion to treat skin blemishes and blotches. In Italy, compresses made from watercress continue to be used to treat arthritis.

In England, as the Industrial Revolution moved people from the leafy shires where they had access to fresh herbs and greens like nettles and goose-grass the year round, watercress beds became a feature of urban sprawl. The most famous was in Hampshire, at the end of the 'watercress railway line' that still helps to keep London supplied with this healthfood.

As an edible herb, watercress is high in vitamin C and a good source of vitamins E and B complex. Rich in iron, it also contains significant amounts of manganese, iodine and calcium (the latter can be absorbed almost as readily from watercress as from milk). It is an excellent antioxidant, protecting the immune system and helping to prevent and treat infections. Homoeopaths use watercress for nervous conditions, constipation and liver disorders. Fresh or dried it is approved for catarrh and other respiratory-tract problems by the German Commission. However, it has been *scientifically* proved only as a remedy for coughs and bronchitis. The latest research indicates that eating watercress may help protect smokers' lungs from the carcinogens present in tobacco and tobacco smoke, as well as possibly protecting against mouth and throat cancers. The herb contains mustard-oil glycosides and nitrites, and its main active constituent as well as the source of its pungency may be its glucosylinate, which is irritating to the mucous membranes, the eyes and skin and yet acts as a counter-irritant by reducing inflammation and mucus in the upper respiratory tract.

Chew your watercress well because pulping down this food medicine releases substantial quantities of isothiocyanates, chemicals containing the poison cyanide. And before you fall down in a faint at this news, let me explain that poisonous they may be in large doses, but some of these naturally occurring isothiocyanates are also effective inhibitors of cancer. Their effects are quite specific, a particular isothiocyanate working on a particular carcinogen. Although most of this work has been carried out on rats, similar results have been observed with smokers who consume watercress. On the basis of these observations about watercress and knowledge of the carcinogenic constituents of cigarette smoke, it appears that a lung-cancer-preventing strategy might well be on the cards.

It is important before consuming this excellent food medicine to be sure of a clean source of supply. It is not recommended during pregnancy, or in cases of gastric or intestinal ulcers or inflammatory kidney disease.

EPHEDRA
Ephedra sinica.
EUROPE AND ASIA

Ephedra, Chinese 'Ma Huang', commonly called 'Joint Pine' is a very ancient plant that is of interest to Botanists and Scientists alike; firstly, as an evolutionary link between flowering plants and conifers and as a medicinal plant. Neither a conifer nor a flowering plant Ephedra produces one of the best anti-congestants. Ephedrine is a sympathetic omimetic amine, resembling adrenaline and amphetamine in its effects. The Neanderthal people of 60,000 years ago didn't know that, but they appear to have made ritual or medical use of it. Various species of Ephedra are now universally called 'Ma Huang', which is an important plant to several traditional natural medicine systems. Ephedra teas have been variously used around the world, from keeping Ghengis Kahn's soldiers awake and as a passive aid to Japanese Zen monks in meditation, to use in an American Mormon tea as a substitute for caffeine. Called 'Whorehouse tea', it was served in brothels in the 1800s in a futile attempt to ward off gonorrhoea and syphilis. The herb is listed in the oldest comprehensive Chinese Materia Medica, Shen Nong Cao Jing, is official in the national pharmacopoeias of China, Germany and Japan and in India, it is listed in the Ayurvedic pharmacopoeia.

Ephedra (E. sinica) has been used since ancient times in China for chills and fevers, coughs, wheezing, asthma, hay fever and is now used by herbalists to treat enuresis, allergies, narcolepsy, and other disorders. However, in Western herbal medicine Ma Huang is used for the onset of colds and flu and more importantly as a treatment for asthma and hay fever.

Ephedra herb contains alkaloids and has the effect of raising blood pressure, to cool fevers and alleviate rheumatism. Among other things, research has shown E. sincia to have anti-viral effects, notably against influenza.

Studied by Chinese Chemists in 1924, ephedrine was synthesised by the German Chemical Firm Merk in 1926 when it began to sweep the market much to the relief of hay fever and asthma sufferers.

The World Health Organization has found the following uses of ephedra preparations to be supported by clinical data: treatment of nasal congestion due to hay fever, allergic rhinitis, acute rhinitis, common cold, sinusitis, and as a brocnchodilator in the treatment of bronchial asthma. It should be noted that the use of dietary supplements that contain ephedra alkaloids may pose a health risk to some persons. Appropriate use of inhalants do not commonly cause serious side effects. However, recent cases of over-the counter accidental overdose and abuse have caused concern and in the UK it is now officially only available for use by medical herbalists.

Ephedra may not be used with Drugs: Oxytocin, Methoyldopa, B-blockers, Caffeine, MAOIs, Theophyline, Sympathomoimetics, St John's wort, Guanethidine and Cardiac glycosides because of potential for increased syjmpathomimetic action, hypertension or CNS stimulation.

15

Feeling a Little Liverish?

Your liver is the heaviest gland in your body, weighing about 1.5 kilograms. It stores carbohydrates as glycogen and detoxifies many waste substances, using the products of this process to synthesise new proteins and change the consistency of fats. It is also a storehouse for vitamins A, D and B_{12}, a warehouse, a breaker's yard, a recycling centre and a factory. Liver is the keystone organ with its own self-structuring and self-repairing systems, whose capabilities, amazing as they are, are not a figment of a *Star Trek* character's imagination; all living things do what you and your liver do, all the time. All this activity uses a lot of energy and produces a lot of heat, but not even this goes to waste, as it helps us keep our bodies up to working temperature.

So what happens when you do feel a little liverish? Fried eggs, bacon and chips may long have been your favourite meal, but all at once the very thought makes you feel more than a little queasy. Suddenly orange juice and even stone fruits turn you off, while itching and/or an insatiable thirst warn you that something is wrong. No wonder you become out of sorts and irritable with everyone and the world in general. 'Feeling a little liverish, old man?' is the last question you want to be asked, but take heed and do something about it before someone does ask! After all, there might be something really wrong – hepatitis, cirrhosis, gallstones or even cancer. So it's off to the doctor for a check-up. And if you get the all-clear but the symptoms persist, then it's probably time for a change of lifestyle. Your liver knows best.

Remember your lymphatic system and the lymph it transports around your body, bathing every living cell? To recap: lymph is a watery fluid composed of blood plasma, and contains white blood cells, which are an important part of your defence system and transport important products and raw materials to and from working cells. Whereas the blood system is the body's long-haul route fast-tracked by the heart, the lymphatic system comprises the much slower short-haul routes, majoring on local deliveries and motivated only by movements in the community of cells round about, especially muscle cells. So to keep the system up and going regular exercise is essential: walking to school or to work is great, while walking the dog makes Fido your lymph's best friend. Then there are all those sports, from jogging to marathons, bowls to squash, swimming to bungy-jumping – whatever takes your fancy, regular exercise *of some sort* is what the lymphatics require. Gardening is great with all the bending and stretching it calls for, e-bends, leg, back and arm exercises all the year round – it's a life-long pastime for you and your lymphatics. And it's official! Recent research shows that gardening is ace when it comes to maintaining general good health. Ballroom dancing is ideal for getting the lymph smoothing along, while the more modern rhythms exercise lymphatics you never knew you had.

Although things are changing rapidly, many people in China still get up early and go through a complex routine of that exercise called t'ai chi. The full workout, which is performed as a community ritual, gently exercises every lymph node known to man or woman. Feeling a bit embarrassed about doing t'ai chi? Well, remember those flowing movements are the very basis of the martial arts. But if you are feeling liverish, especially if you are not used to taking exercise, take it easy as you ease your lymphatics back towards black-belt standard.

In fact, you should never overdo it, and however much you crave fatty meals and alcohol, take it easy in that department too. Cirrhosis afflicts twice as many men as women, and too much alcohol is a prime cause of this complaint. In the long term, the liver can't cope with it pouring through, whether in long bouts or in fits and starts. Bits of it start to die and, although it has remarkable powers of regeneration, who wants to be opened up to facilitate removal of the dead bits?

As movement of the contents of the lymphatic system is naturally slow bacterial attack and infection is much more likely. One reason why the lymph is rich in white blood cells, which congregate in the lymph nodes. Some lymphatic structures like the tonsils and spleen are large, while others are smaller and are found throughout the system. They often swell up and get painful when your body is under attack.

Massage is a very good way of getting at parts of your lymphatic system that other exercises never reach. Aromatherapeutic massage, pioneered in India, is now all the rage in the West – you can even get it on the NHS. Essential oils are rubbed on to the body, and the aim is to knead them deep down into the circulatory system so that their effect is carried to the lymph nodes. And there is good evidence that some of the oils diffuse in, so it isn't just the aroma that makes us feel so good. You arise from the massage table ready for anything – but not, please, another meal swimming in saturated fat.

LYCIUM, CHINESE WOLFBERRY
Lycium chinense

CHINA

Lycium is native to lowland China and is found in Tibet. It is also called Chinese boxthorn, 'discordant matrimony vine', the Duke of Argyll's tea-tree and, commonly, wolfberry. Lycium is a primary Chinese tonic herb; the root bark (*di gu pi*) and fruits (*gou qi zi*) are both used in Chinese medicines. The roots were first mentioned c. 500 AD and its fruits in Shen Nong's *Great Herbal*, compiled in the first century AD. According to legend, the use of lycium together with other tonic herbs allowed one Chinese herbalist to attain an age of over 250 years. Today the herb is very popular in Taiwan, where in the Taipei area alone it is possible to buy twenty medicinal materials derived from lycium. Its legendary energising tonic power for longevity has become so popular that Ningxia, known as the home town of Chinese wolfberry, produced 103 tonnes of its juice for export to the United States during May–December 2001.

On the strength of clinical tests, Chinese medical experts say that wolfberries produced in the Ningxia region make an excellent tonic that helps promote and adjust the functions of the immune system, protects the liver and prolongs life. The spotlight is also trained on the wolfberry's nutritional value: it contains more beta-carotene than carrots, 19 amino acids, 21 trace minerals and 31 per cent polysaccharides. All over China, 'tea attendants' are a common sight in restaurants serving *gou qi zi* tea to diners, and wolfberries are eaten like raisins. Traditional Chinese

herbalists use lycium's bright-red berries to improve the circulation and to tone and protect the liver and kidneys. The root is
used to lower blood pressure and blood cholesterol. In America
the fruit is incorporated into supplements to boost the immune
system and to counteract ageing, and used in fitness capsules,
snacks, teas and even eye and wrinkle creams.

Lycium fruits contain betaine, copper, iron, magnesium, zeaxanthin and zinc, and the leaves some vitamin E. Scientific
research now confirms that the berries protect the liver from
damage caused by environmental toxins: in particular, the compound zeaxanthin diplamitate protects it against carbon tetra-
chloride toxicity. Korean research in 2002 has also found that
ZD, a carotenoid, effectively inhibits hepatic fibrosis in rats,
which may partly be because it is antioxidant. It has also been
shown that the wolfberry root stimulates the involuntary nervous
system governing the internal organs and relaxes artery walls,
allowing them to expand and thus lowering blood pressure. As a
result, the root is beginning to be used in China to treat high
blood pressure. In Chinese medicine it is credited with improving
vision, and a tea mixed with chrysanthemum is used for hangovers – another warning of liver problems on the horizon.

Do not take wolfberry if you have an inflammatory condition,
poor digestion or a tendency to bloating. Recent research also
suggests that the anticoagulant drug warfarin should not be taken
at the same time as wolfberry.

CHIRATA, CHIRAYATA
Swertia chirata
NORTHERN INDIA, NEPAL

Chirata grows wild throughout the pastures and slopes of the
Himalayas and also occurs in mountainous regions of North
America, Eurasia and Africa. Chirata or *kirata-tikta*, which means
'bitter plant', is a gentian-like herb with digestive properties that
is used in traditional Ayurvedic medicine to treat *pitta* (meaning
'fire') conditions – that is, conditions involving fever. It is held in

considerable esteem by the Hindus. The name *S. chirata* is used of many gentian-type plants sold in Indian bazaars. True chirata has yellowish pith, is extremely bitter and has no smell. Chirata is the name of an Indian region, and it was the export of the plant's bitter extract that led to its use in Britain.

The herb acts well on the liver and promotes the secretion of bile, cures constipation and is useful for dyspepsia. It also restores tone after illnesses and, like most bitters, reduces fevers. Chirata BP, usually given as an infusion, is tannin-free and has the added advantage of being prescribed with iron. The main active ingredients are bitters, among which are oxygenated xanthones, which Indian research has shown to be active against both malaria and tuberculosis.

In May 2001 research on several chirata species revealed their ability to fight toxins in cultures of rat hepatocytes, including both tetrachloride- and paracetamol-induced toxicity. Recent research suggests that the non-bitter components of chirata have a broader protective effect on the liver. The plant is antioxidant and, in line with its traditional use, research shows it to be anti-malarial. In a Chinese and Nepalese joint venture, chirata tablets and capsules for liver and kidney diseases are being researched and developed. One of chirata's constituents, amarogentin, the bitterest yet found, is also being studied in South Africa to assess its ability to relieve problems caused by *Leishmania donovani*, a parasite found within the cells of the lymphatic system, spleen and bone marrow.

GREEN TEA
Camellia sinensis

ASIA

Tea was introduced into Europe in the seventeenth century and is now drunk in nearly every country in the world. The most important species, green tea (*C. sinensis*), comes from the same plant as black and oolong teas, but, unlike black tea, the leaves remain unfermented. Unfermented green tea is produced in

China and Japan; black tea comes from India, Sri Lanka and Kenya. Tea is also cultivated in Indonesia, Turkey, Malawi, Pakistan and Argentina. But there is more to this refreshing drink than a good 'cuppa'.

In China, tea has been used both as a drink and as a medicine for approximately five thousand years. In Asian medicine, tea is used to treat heart pain, dizziness, haemorrhoids, headache, excessive thirst, indigestion and drowsiness. Homoeopaths recommend it for headache, heart conditions and insomnia. Research is beginning to show that a cuppa really is a good way of soothing tense, nervous headaches, since the caffeine in tea (and coffee) can provide for the majority of people a 'low but very real level of effectiveness in treating tension-type headaches' and can boost the effectiveness of standard pain-killers. It can also act as quickly as many pain-killing medications.

Contemporary science has also shown that green tea can protect the liver against a variety of toxins, including industrial solvents and alcohol. One of the polyphenols present in a constituent of tea, catechin (trade name Catergen), is a powerful antioxidant, and in part responsible for green tea's liver-protecting properties. In one study of twelve persons with chronic hepatitis B, treatment using Catergen resulted in four experiencing clinically significant improvement; while in animal studies of viral hepatitis, pre-treatment with green tea extract has shown a significant preventive effect.

It is now thought that tea-drinking helps protect against 'slippage' of DNA molecules, which can cause genes to be copied incorrectly, with dangerous results that are known to cause cancer. Both green and black teas' antioxidants are thought to help reduce the risk of certain cancers, such as gastrointestinal, stomach, colon and 'potentially' breast cancer. The main active constituents of green tea are polyphenols, and the flavonol epigallocarchehin-gallate can inhibit the development of malignant brain tumours. The polyphenols in green tea extract are also preventive antioxidants for the heart and a potential aid after heart attacks, as well as offering protection against ultraviolet injury, sunburn and even skin cancer. Furthermore, green tea may prove to be a boon in the obesity boom, as an appetite suppressant, to encourage and maintain weight loss.

Be aware that the caffeine in teas may cause stimulation and increase the stimulatory effects of theophyline and xanthine derivatives, while increasing the levels of lithium or of products containing caffeine concentrations, e.g. guarana (see p. 000). (Guarana is a caffeine-rich drink made from the guarana seeds that grow in Brazil.)

ARTICHOKE
Cynara scolymus
MEDITERRANEAN

The artichoke has been a diner's delight since the time of the ancient Greeks. It has been used as a herbal remedy since the fourth century BC, and there is mention of the plant in Greek and Roman literature since 77 AD. Cultivated by the Moors near Granada, Spain, around 800, it had been introduced to Europe from North Africa by the Greeks, and was subsequently used as an aid to digestion by the Romans and the French. The artichoke didn't make it to England till about 1548, and it went to America with the Spanish settlers of California where it is now grown in vast quantities.

Traditionally, artichoke was used for dyspepsia or indigestion. Bitter and slightly salty, as a herb it is now used to alleviate chronic liver and gall-bladder diseases and to treat arteriosclerosis and diabetes. It has been shown that artichoke reduces cholesterol levels and helps metabolise fats. As a herb, it is mainly used to protect the liver and to stimulate its function. The head, leaves and heart are an excellent source of folate and potassium and, as the root of the plant does not contain many of its active ingredients, eating the 'globe' makes a very efficacious entrée.

Do not eat artichoke if you are suffering from a bile-duct blockage, as it stimulates the flow of bile. Use it with caution if you suffer from gallstones, as it could cause painful spasms. For some, frequent contact with the plant can lead to allergic reactions.

Despite its name the Jerusalem artichoke, a root crop discovered and developed by the Americas' native peoples, is a member of the daisy flower family.

MILKTHISTLE
Silybum marianum.

Today, many people's livers have a lot to put up with: a daily burden of alcohol, fast food, traffic emissions, environmental chemicals, prescription pill-popping.

Unfortunately a damaged liver will get short shrift from conventional medicine; there's little on offer except powerful steroids and as a last gasp option a liver transplant. Milkthistle is a wonderful weed that can help the liver cope. Found throughout the Mediterranean and at altitude in eastern Africa, the herb was known to Dioscorides in the 1st century AD and Pliny the Roman naturalist recommended it. Traditionally, it has long been used in the UK to stimulate bile production and to detoxify the liver. It gathered momentum in allopathic medicine and is contained in various brands of proprietary medicine for the treatment of liver ailments. It is also used in homoeopathy for hepatic disorders. Herbalists also used the herb for nursing mothers, as a bitter tonic and as an antidepressant in addition to liver complaints.

More recently herbalists had been using the herb in line with the revelations of modern research. In it's revisited modern usage, milkthistle is still employed as a bitter and diuretic tonic and is scientifically known to help regenerate liver cells, stimulate bile flow and aid liver and gall bladder diseases and complaints such as jaundice. Milkthistle contains a complex of flavolignans called 'Silymarin'. Silymarin extracted from Milkthistle seeds has been found to have a highly liver-protective effect, helping to maintain liver function and prevent damage. It is also used to counteract the effects of the over consumption of alcohol, against drug-abuse, liver damage and as an antidote to fungal poisoning. Although only rare case reports of gastrointestinal disturbances and allergic skin rashes have been published, recent research indicates that the flavonoid content and free radical scavenging properties. Experiments of this herb show great promise

In Germany, research has confirmed that silymarin is successful to treat hepatitis and cirrhosis of the liver. Science has proved silymarin can help reconstruct damaged liver cells in cases of alcohol poisoning. It helps heal hepatitis B, but its use should be declared to your health provider. There is also anecdotal evidence of the sudden disappearance of inoperable liver cancer.

16

Coming to Your Senses

Taste, smell, touch, hearing and sight – these are the five senses with which we test the environment around us. Asked that age-old question 'Which one you would most readily give up?', the age-old answer is a long pause for thought. After a lot of thought I can list mine in ascending order: I think I would, if I had to, relinquish the power of taste first, then smell, hearing, touch and last, sight. There is perhaps a sixth called 'the sense of health': complex it may be, but our sense of health monitors our environment. Our health is a barometer for the whole environment upon which we depend and of which we are a part. We are what we eat and what the rest of our environment allows us to be. This sixth sense is the subject of this book.

We can in the main distinguish only four *tastes*: sweet, salty, sour and bitter. Different parts of our tongues show different sensitivities to each: bitter at the back, hence the aftertaste of a real pint; sweetness at the tip, ideal for testing that lollipop; salty and sour along the edge.

Substances like ginger and chocolate are good at masking other tastes. Gingerbread was invented to use up mouldy flour in the days before sell-by dates, and cranberry and mint sauce used to help mouldy meat on its way towards further digestion. Salt, a preservative, has become the flavour-enhancer and thirst-maker in crisps; and monosodium glutamate, originally extracted from seaweed, now finds its way into most processed foods. Research using pure chemicals is showing that there are other tastes, and individuals sometimes differ greatly in sensitivity to them. Whisky-blenders, it would seem, are born, not made, and much of their acuity, as with appreciating food, depends on the sense of *smell* – nose, not tongue.

Complex as our nasal passages may be, the bit that allows us to savour the multitude of volatile substances that get up our noses, situated high up inside each nostril, covers only some 2.5 square centimetres. That's why a good long sniff helps a lot. The human nose reacts to the aroma of the active principle in garlic at almost homoeopathic concentrations, so no wonder she or he can smell it on your breath. Fantastic, but that still means that for each square centimetre of the receptive patches around 30,000 million molecules of the chemical per second have got up your nose. Thank goodness water doesn't have a smell, because even at freezing point each cubic centimetre of air contains 1,500 billion water molecules. Many animals, including insects, are said to be much better at smelling than we are, reacting to just a few molecules of an attractant produced downwind by a potential mate. These special volatile messengers are called 'pheromones'. How important are they in attracting us across a crowded room and turning us on at closer range? Our brains don't respond by commenting, 'What a nice smell' – perhaps we don't smell them in the strict sense of the word. It is more direct than that: it simply gets us, or parts of us, moving. Perhaps water does have a smell; it just doesn't tickle your fancy.

Recent research suggests that all those dead cells that fall from our skin every day get carried up to other special organs high in our nostrils: pits well supplied with bristle-like sensory hairs, first described by Ludwig Jacobsen in 1809, that respond not to aromas but to chemicals on those skin cells that waft from our bodies every day. Forty million love darts – perhaps this is the real meaning of sharing skin – dating back to our reptilian days, long before Eve's exploits in the Garden of Eden. Human pheromones? Well, some are already on the market, or so says the perfume industry.

Another important aspect of your smell faculty, or olfaction, is that your nose gets tired or, to be exact, your sense of smell becomes fatigued and switches off. Have you ever wondered where the smell of old sweat goes after you have been in a gymnasium for a few minutes, or how people live with their own halitosis? Most of our senses appear to work in this way: they sense the difference between two states, but they soon get tired. We can feel the difference between hot and cold, for instance: our skin has thousands of tiny warmth receptors and thousands of tiny cold receptors. They don't work in absolute terms like a thermometer, but they register differences, changes as little as 0.001 degree per second – sensitive you! We are also sensitive to *touch* and *pain*; both have specific receptors in the skin, but when does touch become pressure and pressure become pain? Each appears to have a threshold, and that threshold differs between individuals. Hairs, even cats' whiskers, are themselves insensitive to touch; when acted upon by an outside force – when they brush past your leg, for example – they simply rock the receptors around their base.

Pain itself is a somewhat subjective phenomenon. Soldiers engaged in war ask for many fewer sedatives than civilians suffering from comparable wounds. We are in many ways taught to feel pain via warnings such as 'This may hurt a little', 'Be careful – you may get hurt.' Dogs raised in conditions where they are shielded from harmful stimulation have been shown to grow up almost unaware of pain. What is more, once we have learned about pain we use it to communicate, and in most cases to get our own way. Sweeties are one of the most effective analgesics for children, and dental surgeons use pleasant sound to damp down our aversion to the noise of the drill. Researchers have found that when wearing earphones supplied with steady Muzak plus 'white noise', the level of which they could adjust, 650 out of 1,000 dental patients felt no pain, while 250 asked for no other pain-killer. Either it worked, or it was only 10 per cent that were not lying through their teeth.

It is very hard to imagine what it would be like to live in a completely silent world, almost as hard as explaining sight to a person who has been blind since birth. The ear is an amazing organ that allows us to discriminate between around 340,000 different tones. *Hearing*, both at the top and at the bottom end of the range, appears to merge with the sense of touch. Top notes hurt, the lowest make us shudder, very loud noise damages our sense of hearing permanently. So go easy on the control knob, however much the dentist's drill hurts: heavy metal could be doing you acoustic harm.

Our ears not only tell us where we are in relation to other noisy things, but they also allow us to orientate ourselves in relation to the hidden force of gravity. Plants can do it, for their shoots always turn away from, and their roots towards, the force of gravity. We can see other things reacting to gravity – as in the case of Isaac Newton, we can feel an apple fall on our heads. However, our main sense of position in relation (1) to the force of gravity and (2) to change of direction and speed is located in our ears' semicircular canals. The first relates to two little bulbs that contain sensitive cells with a tuft of hairs supporting a tiny pebble of 'chalk', free to roll about telling us which is up and which is down. The second relates to three canals set almost at right-angles to each other, full of fluid that swirls around as we move about in our own three-dimensional space. Groups of sensory cells, each again supplied with tufts of hair, pick up the swirling motion, thereby allowing us to orientate and even making us feel dizzy or sick.

Always remember that ageing is going to take away the top notes, while the likelihood of tinnitus – ringing, roaring or hissing in the ears – also increases in old age. Research indicates that the brain 'cycles' certain sounds that indicate danger, then turns up their volume little by little until these annoying and in some cases debilitating noises are established.

The fact that we can *see* at all depends on nerve receptors, the rods and cones that make up the retinas of our eyes. The cones work in bright light, allowing us to see colour and fine detail. The rods work in dim light, letting us perceive images in black and white. The way both work depends on the production of a pigment called 'visual purple'. Visual purple is unstable in the presence of light and breaks down into protein and retinene; the latter further decomposes into vitamin A (a great dietary source of which is carrot).

A 'sight for sore eyes' may seem a rather old-fashioned expression in this day and age, but sore eyes are not a thing of the past. Dickensian tales of seamstresses and others toiling long hours in crowded and poorly lit conditions should have faded with the Factory Act and the arrival of electricity; but unfortunately, electricity has brought another lifestyle complication. Gone are the days when twilight signalled the end of the waking day and nights were at least eight hours long. Now in the incandescent glare we continue to work or to play. That book at bedtime has become Pokemon; channels are being switched twenty-fours hours of the electronic day. Your poor eyes, young or old, are processing twenty-five images each second – it's no wonder sore eyes are an ever commoner sight.

A very visible eye problem, especially among old people, is cataracts. Research shows that triggers to cataract formation include glutathione deficiency, which contributes to a faulty antioxidant defence system within the lens of the eye. Cataract patients also tend to be deficient in vitamin A and the carotenes, lutein and zeaxanthin. Nutrients that can be taken to increase glutathione levels include lipoic acid, vitamins E and C and selenium. Others that may help prevent cataracts include riboflavin (vitamin B_2), pantethine, a derivative of pantothenic acid (vitamin B_5), folic acid, melatonin and plant flavonoids, particularly quercetin and its derivatives.

Another, not so visible, affliction of old age is glaucoma, in which pressure builds up inside the eyeball. Some patients maintain normal intra-ocular pressure, but either way poor circulation results in damage to the optic nerve. As with patients suffering from cataracts, those with glaucoma typically have an inadequate antioxidant defence system, allowing free radicles to do their worst. Some of the herbs mentioned elsewhere have in this book been shown to help. *Ginkgo biloba* (see p. 000) increases circulation to the optic nerve; forskolin, an extract of coleus (*Coleus forskohlii*), has been used topically to lower pressure in the eye; intramuscular injections of red sage (*Salvia miltiorhiza*) have improved visual acuity and peripheral vision in people with glaucoma. This painful condition accounts for 15 per cent of all cases of blindness in the USA. If your eyeballs hurt, please go straight to the doctor for a check-up.

Colour-blindness is much more common in men than in women, and is a genetic condition with as yet no cure in sight. Regular check-ups by your optician can put your mind at ease.

All these vital senses depend on nerve cells, so again we return to the subject of those essential unsaturated fatty acids. As our bodies can't make them, we must get them from the food we eat. Every day of our lives we need sufficient linoleic and alpha-linolenic acid in our diets: the natural source of the former is seeds, nuts and whole grains; the latter is found in leaves, fish and shellfish. However, there is a problem, for even these acids can be too saturated with hydrogen to do the job we need them to do, and so our bodies have to go to all the trouble of further desaturation and processing. And I must say it again: when it comes to maintaining the balance, our Western diets oozing with saturates are of no help at all.

A mere hundred years ago our diets had hardly changed since the Stone Age; the processed-food revolution was yet to come. Metabolically we were and still are in effect hunter-gatherers; dietwise our bodies are still, in the main, programmed to deal with a great diversity of meat, fish and veg. Although we retain into adulthood the ability to digest lactose, the main energy store in our mothers' milk, our digestive systems still expect to be fed on wholefoods. Fruit and vegetables from early spring until autumn; grains, fruits and nuts in summer and autumn, with fish, shellfish and game whenever available. Nutritional scientists have calculated the make-up of the diet of Palaeolithic people, the diet our bodies are still programmed to thrive on. Compare it with the diet of today:

	Palaeolithic diet	Present-day diet
protein (g)	34	15
carbohydrate (g)	45	42
fat (g)	21	38
fibre (g)	46	21
sodium (mg)	690	2,800
calcium (mg)	1,580	780
ascorbic acid (mg)	392	64

Perhaps most importantly, the ratio of polyunsaturated to saturated fat was 1.41 then and is 0.39 now. Things have certainly changed, and much of that change has taken place since the end of the Second World War, when the war on our health and our environment started on the home front with two well disguised secret weapons: intensive agriculture and food processing.

Dr Stephen Davies, from whose work I have borrowed the above figures, has summarised the factors that may influence the nutrient content and availability of nutrients in our modern food supply. The list gets longer as the packets get bigger to accommodate all the information. Much of this consists of novel chemicals, and although in the main they have been tested for toxicity, carcinogenicity and allergic reaction, their long-term effects on the bioavailability of nutrients, let alone on their (or our) genes, are unknown. Official figures tell us that already more than 3,794 such additives are in circulation in the British diet. Be that as it may, the vital differences between our diet and that of our Stone Age ancestors appear to be:

 * Too much refined sugar, which is linked with tooth decay, blood-sugar upsets and obesity.

* Too much saturated fat in relation to those essential polyunsat-urates, which is linked with heart attack, stroke, arthritis, prostate and liver problems.
* Too little roughage, linked with bowel problems.
* Too much polished grain, making the back of the cereal pack-et look like an advert for food additives.
* Too little ascorbic acid, perhaps reducing resistance to infec-tions such as the common cold.
* Too much alcohol and caffeine, exacerbating many of the above.
* *Nicotiana tabacum* – to clarify – the smoking of this now dread-ed weed.

Believe it or not, these chemical changes, small though they may be on the grand scale of things, can affect our basic senses. Ponder the fact that the Danes, in need of foreign currency after the First World War, exported all their butter, so the locals had to make do on mar-garine. The result: a high incidence of blindness among Danish chil-dren.

CARROT
Daucus carota
AFGHANISTAN, CENTRAL ASIA

Carrots help you to see in the dark – true or false? Well, it's true; along with green vegetables and liver, they contain beta-carotene, which our bodies turn into vitamin A (also called retinol), which is absolutely essential for vision in general and night blindness in particular. Despite the fact that cats have much better night vision than we do, they can't perform this chemical trick. Of course, they don't need to because being carnivores they get all the vita-min A they need from the prey they eat.

Neolithic people consumed the wild carrot over seven thou-sand years ago and temple drawings dating from around 2000 BC show that it was an important plant in Egypt, a major producer of carrot-seed oil today. Carrots were originally purple, and only became orange after patriotic sixteenth-century Dutch farmers developed the colour, probably from mutant seed imported from North Africa.

Young raw domestic carrot root is highly nutritious, containing that all-important precursor of retinol as well as many other vitamins and folic acid. At the University of Wisconsin 'beta-3' carrots are being bred to yield three to five times more carotenes than normal, ready to help countries where severe vitamin A deficiency leaves hundreds of thousand of people blind each year.

The recent back-to-basics revival of the purple carrot is also good news, for not only does the ancient pigment contain over twice as much alpha- and beta-carotenes than the modern breed, but it also contains antioxidant, anticarcinogenic anthocyanins. A diet rich in carotenes can also help ward off age-related degenerative diseases such as arthritis and heart disease.

Puréed raw carrots provide more bioavailable alpha- and beta-carotenes than boiled and mashed ones, which is good news for babies, while carrot chips are also a good way to administer their goodness to anti-carrot kids. Together with lycopene, carrots can boost the vitamin A and iron intake of lactating women and help bolster both pre- and postmenopausal women against ovarian cancer. A serving of carrots when consuming spreads containing sterol or stanol esters maintains the carotene content of blood plasma while significantly lowering LDL-cholesterol concentrations. In Poland, researchers have found that consuming carrots at least three times a week substantially lowers the risk of lung cancer developing in women. It is, however, possible to overdose on beta-carotene, causing yellowy-orange skin discoloration, so carotenes are best eaten with other fruits and vegetables.

MAIDENHAIR TREE
Ginkgo biloba

CHINA

Ginkgo, the fruits and leaves of which were eaten by dinosaurs, is showing some promising results in treating hearing disorders.

More than any of our other sense organs, our ears get us into trouble and cause us the most problems. One reason for this is that they also perform another crucially important function: that of balance.

Although antibiotics have done much to alleviate the once dreaded mastoid infections of the middle ear, they are unfortunately far from uncommon in these days of polluted waters, scuba addicts being especially at risk. If disease destroyed both your inner ears, not only would you be totally deaf, but also your ability to balance would be at issue. If you have bad earache, for any reason, go straight to the doctor – your ears are warning you.

Although there are dissenters, most scientists agree that the use of *Ginkgo biloba* extract as a vasodilator of the cochlea, or inner ear, may be beneficial in tinnitus treatment. Short-standing disorders have a better prognosis, so that better results can be expected with early-onset treatment. German research has found that *G. biloba* extract administered orally in cases of sudden idiopathic hearing loss, especially where neither tinnitus nor vertigo are present, appears to speed up the recovery of patients so that they are better within one week and stand a good chance of recovering completely. Ginkgo has been shown to be as effective as treatment with Pentoxifylline, a proprietary drug.

BREWER'S YEAST
Saccharomyces cerevisiae
WORLDWIDE

Yeast microbes are probably one of the earliest domesticated organisms. Yeast was also the first food additive, for its spores are always blowing about on the wind and will latch on to any store of sugar. People have used yeast for fermentation and baking throughout history. One of the first references to its medical use comes in the Ebers papyrus, written c. 1500 BC, which recommends yeast as a cure for constipation. Brewer's yeast is considered a good diet supplement because it has a lot of nutrients packed into a small volume and is almost predigested. This 'phytofood' is also a commercial source of proteins and of the vitamin B complex. Yeast extract, as well as the yeast used in baking and brewing (called 'God is good' up to the late 1700s), helps keep the metabolism, the nervous system and the body tissues in good health. It also contains folate, needed for blood-cell formation, and various minerals including potassium, magnesium and zinc. Some yeasts are cultured in chromium-containing media and absorb that mineral, making it bioavailable. (Chromium is a vital link in the chain that makes glucose available to the body, which is particularly important to diabetics.)

The medicinal applications of brewer's yeast relate to the treatment of acute diarrhoea, the prevention of candida, the treatment of acne and the alleviation of mild pre-menstrual syndrome (PMS). It is used for disorders associated with specific diseases, such as botulism, blackleg, tetanus and gas gangrene, which are caused by the organism clostridium, which is pathogenic to both people and animals. It is also being investigated for treating candida in children with cystic fibrosis. Brewer's yeast can inhibit the growth (in vitro) of many potentially pathogenic organisms.

Yeast-derived fibre is a more concentrated source of beta-glucan than the average oat product and is being tested in a wide variety of food products. Beta-glucan, a natural chemical extracted from yeast (and plant) cell walls, is an immune-system booster with enormous potential in combating cancer, AIDS, surgical infection and even the effects of radiation. Medicinal brewer's yeast is a focus of ongoing medical and scientific investigation. It is one of only a handful of microbes on earth whose unique gene script has recently been comprehensively deciphered. NASA fully expects that some kind of life-form similar to yeast will be found on other planets.

17

You'll Be a Man, My Son

It was all your dad's fault. The die was cast about twenty-one months before your first birthday as a sperm and an egg became one – a new and unique individual, planted somewhere very special, safe inside your mum.

The egg contained a library of genetic information, arranged in twenty-three floppy lists called chromosomes. Enough to make your mum exactly what she was or is: Wimbledon champion or housewife from Wapping. The sperm, though only one seventy-five-thousandth the size of the egg, contained a similar library of information. Enough to make Dad exactly the way he was or is: chief executive or top of the pops. Chance had already played its trump card. Usually a mum produces only one egg at a time, each one unique. Dad, on the other hand, produces around 400 million sperm, more than enough to father the whole population of the USA at each ejaculation. Each sperm contains a unique set of genes, an outboard motor and an inbuilt sense of direction and purpose: Find that Egg and Fertilise It.

So it set off on the race of its and your life, a race which, in comparative terms, is a bit like you or me swimming eight miles, and uphill all the way. What is more, about 399,999,999 unlucky sperm died in the ascent, all so as to make individual, brilliant, scintillating You. Think, next time you use a condom – and I hope you do, unless you and your partner are using another form of contraceptive or are planning to enlarge your family – of all those poor unsuccessful sperm banging their little heads against the wall. (It's a good thing it's made of rubber.)

Not all sperm are perfect; in fact, about 10 per cent of them come in all sorts of malformed shapes and sizes. For a long time these were thought to perform no useful function; so why should the male of the species have wasted all the raw materials used in their manufacture? Recent research has indicated that they may play a rather strange role.

They are probably kamikaze sperm whose sole object in their short life is to attack and destroy any perfect sperm derived from another male. This theory opens up all sorts of intriguing possibilities, the most likely of which suggests that monogamy was only a relatively recent development in the human race. Polyandrous women were indeed the norm among some tribal people. It would have been in those situations that the kamikaze sperms would have come into their own, battling it out in the struggle for the survival of the fittest and for the one who was to become a dad.

Be that as it may, in the data set you received there was an X chromosome from your mum (eggs only have X chromosomes) and a Y chromosome from your dad (sperms can have X or Y). XY makes for a male and XX for a female.

The next seven days were crucial in your development and, just as for the rest of your life, environment played a very important role. At this particular juncture you were a bonny ball of cells, safely embedded in the wall of your mum's uterus: your environment for the next nine months, suffused with a balanced supply of those all-important brain-building unsaturated fatty acids and a balanced mixture of male and female hormones. Too many female hormones, and on day seven your maleness would have been put in jeopardy and six weeks later your male organs would not have started to form. So it all comes down to hormones, and herein lies one of the strangest facts of life.

There may not be much difference in chemical terms between the male and the female hormone, but it's enough to make all the difference to you.

From that point on in your life were laid down the first cells that would multiply and eventually give rise to your testes, and ever after, those cells took on a central role in your male control system. They started to produce your very own male hormones, so helping to keep the whole you in balance and at the peak of male perfection. Despite the fact that you probably don't fill each unforgiving minute with sixty seconds' worth of distance run, that's nonetheless how you got the way you are – a man, my son.

One last word on sex and gender. In recent years concern has been increasing over the use in the oral contraceptive of sex hormones synthesised from plants, a development that has revolutionised both family planning and, some suggest, sexual behaviour. Sex and other growth hormones are also used in the raising of farm animals, potentially mucking up the natural balance of male and female hormones in our environment; for remember – we are what we eat. These facts certainly counsel for an organic diet during pregnancy.

CATUABA
Trichillia catigua
BRAZIL, CENTRAL AMERICA

'Out of this world' best describes this amazing Brazilian rainforest herb that was discovered by the Tupi-Guarani people of the Amazon rainforest and has been used by them for over five hundred years. They composed many songs singing its praises: for instance, one that goes, 'If a man becomes a father up to sixty it was him. If he's older than sixty it was catuaba.' It is said that catuaba, also called 'the good tree', leads first to erotic dreams, then to increased libido. It grows in northern Brazil and Central America. Today, backed by Brazilian government investigations, catuaba is used in diverse forms in products around the world, including whole herbs, as a herbal extract in powdered or liquid form, as a tincture, a decoction, a tea, as capsules and as 'wild catuaba exotic sweet red wine', for herbal-medicinal purposes.

In Brazilian herbal medicine catuaba bark, which regrows after it is removed from the tree, is considered mainly as a stimulant and tonic for the central nervous system, while being valued for its aphrodisiac properties. It also improves mood and promotes restful sleep. A decoction is used for sexual impotence in both men and women, although the best results reported are for male impotence. It is helpful in cases of agitation, nervousness, neurasthenia, and failing memory, as well as many other kinds of nervous condition such as insomnia, hypochondria and neurological pain; and in Peru it is used against skin cancer.

Currently sold as a dietary supplement in France, Germany and the USA, in Europe the herb is considered an aphrodisiac and a brain and nerve stimulant. Bark 'tea' is used for sexual frailty, impotence, nervous exhaustion and general debility. In America, the tea is used as a tonic for the genitals and as a stimulant for impotence and general fatigue or depletion; it is also found to be effective in America in cases of hypertension-related insomnia, nervous disorder and poor recall.

Related to plants that are sources of cocaine, catuaba contains none of the active cocaine alkaloids and has produced no evidence of side-effects, even after long-term use. It constituents include flavonoids, saponins, alkaloids, tannins, aromatic oils and fatty resins, and minerals including calcium and magnesium. Catuaba also contains three alkaloids dubbed catuabine A, B and C that are believed to enhance sexual function by stimulating the nervous system.

MALE GEAR AND ALL THAT JAZZ

The testis Please note that the correct terms are 'testis' and 'testes' (plural), for 'testicle' is the diminutive of the word and means 'very small' – yours may be, but I will use the correct term all the same. Big or small, testes not only produce a regular supply of male hormones, but all those sperm and some of the seminal fluid in which they swim. Unless ejaculation opens up the escape route, all will be broken down and the raw materials reabsorbed ready for reuse. Recycling has always played a key part in the survival of the fittest.

Testes dangling unprotected in the scrotum may not seem or feel such a good arrangement, especially if you get kicked in the wrong place. So why has evolution made us well hung *and* unprotected? The problem is that spermatogenesis, the production of sperm, comes to a halt at body temperature, so in the absence of an inbuilt cooling system they have to dangle in order to stay real cool. Beware all those in the habit of wearing tight jeans and even tighter pants. Nudity was the original answer, and Scotsmen are traditionally OK, while good old baggy underpants like Dad used to wear still make good sense. Horses, tigers and the fastest of all, cheetahs, have the ability to winch them up while on the run, and squirrels do so when fighting because they have the nasty habit of biting their oponent below the belt. Martial arts experts can apparently train themselves to do the same, although I have never seen any statistics regarding their love life.

'Cryptorchidism' describes the condition in which the testes don't descend. Untreated or untreatable, the result is no sperm and hence sterility. However, under normal circumstances, at a given time dependent upon those hormones and differing from individual to individual, they will descend down the inguinal canals and out into the cool and be thus able to begin their lifelong work: the manufacture of an incredible 500 billion sperm in your lifetime. That is over 250 per heart-throb.

The penis You may call yours Willy or some other pet name, and you will probably boast about its size while being amazed at the way it shrinks in the cold and rises to the occasion. Nature ordained that the ultra-sensitive tip or, to give it its proper name, glans penis, be covered with a sheath of skin. However, a number of tribes, cults and religions, especially in the dry tropics and subtropics, ordain the ritual removal of this sheath of skin by circumcision. For a long time there was no proof or indication that this practice, barbaric to some, either improves or impairs the standing of the member or the health of its owner, as long as normal levels of hygiene are maintained.

Nevertheless, in the dry tropics where water for regular washing can be a luxury, circumcision does make sense. In the absence of sufficient water, hands may be cleansed with dry sand before a meal; but it would take true grit to give your penis such a ritual scrub after a pee. The importance of penal cleansing was highlighted recently in relation to certain parts of Africa where plantains (cooking bananas) have become a profitable export crop and hence a new local staple. Unfortunately, plantains contain substances that can be changed into carcinogens once inside the body. The body does its best to get rid of them via the urine, but the problem is (or was) that tiny amounts trapped under the foreskin can become concentrated enough to initiate a very inconvenient form of cancer.

The shaft of the penis is made of erectile tissue, which means it can be engorged with blood (this happens when the blood's escape route back to the veins is temporarily shut off). Various forms of stimulation can arouse erection, and recovery after ejaculation takes at least seven minutes – and that's a record.

The epididymides and gubernacula No, I am not gibbering. Epididymides are small sacs, which can store four ejaculations' worth of sperm ready for use. And I bet you didn't know you had two gubernacula (singular: gubernaculum), but I bet you are glad you have. They act as shock-absorbers, independent suspension to your own particular load of balls.

The urethra This is the escape route for both sperm and urine.

The prostate As you get old you will probably wish that you didn't have such a thing, for the prostate is one of the major causes of premature death in older gentlemen, especially in the developed world. It's a chestnut-sized gland that sits at the neck of your bladder. Its sole purpose appears to be to secrete an alkaline addition to the seminal fluid. Although it alters in size naturally, problems arise if it gets so big that it presses against your urethra, slowing or even stopping the flow of urine. This is very painful and, if untreated, could lead to death by poisoning as toxic substances accumulate in your body.

The commonest condition that can cause all this to happen is benign prostatic hyperplasia (BPH). If you are over forty, then you have either got it or you will have a male friend who does. This non-infectious, non-malignant enlargement of the prostate appears to be among the major problems of growing old. Most of us will suffer no more than a little discomfort and urgency. However, if the symptoms appear to persist or worsen, reassure yourself and go to your doctor. In the USA hospital treatment and surgery for this syndrome cost in excess of a billion dollars a year. There is even an International Prostate Symptoms Score (IPSS), or 'I can't PISS', as the case may be, to help you make up your mind that a visit to the doctor is worth while. The symptoms it lists are as follows – check them out and see how you score.

* Have you got a weak urinary stream?
* Do you have to push or strain to begin urinating?
* Do you experience a sensation of not having completely emptied your bladder after urinating?
* Do you need to go again within two hours of urinating?
* Do you stop and start again during urination?
* Do you find it difficult to postpone urination?
* Do you have to get up to urinate between going to bed and getting up in the morning?

All of you will know that a number of these so-called symptoms can be turned on and off by lifestyle factors, such as when and how much you do or don't drink, and whether you are a regular or irregular bedtimer or getter-upper. There is also the schoolboy's own way of testing the strength of your urine stream. But seeing how far you can pee up the urinal wall is not so hygienic in these days of diddy-bowls (though still possible if you can find one of those magnificent Victorian loo emporia – then perhaps you could do the Old Grey Whistle Test in a fitting environment). Anyway, if these things persist and you are tempted to say 'Why bother?', please consider the following facts.

The embarrassing symptoms of BPH can have a drastic effect on your life. Common complaints are having to avoid drinking at certain times, having to reduce total fluid intake, having to discover in advance whether there are toilets in places you want to visit, not taking part in social and leisure activities because of embarrassment. And how about your sex life? A recent Mori poll of eight hundred men over the age of fifty showed that almost half had experienced poor sex drive and erection or ejaculatory problems over the past year. Twenty per cent of those with symptoms of BPH had sex at least once a week compared with 40 per cent of men without symptoms, and men with two or more symptoms of prostatism would have liked to have sex more often than their symptoms allowed.

Which club do you want to join?

Prostatitis, inflammation of the prostate gland, is a much less common affliction than those listed so far, and can develop in one of three forms: acute bacterial, chronic bacterial or non-bacterial, which is caused by malfunction of the waterworks. Symptoms of all three are low back pain, especially after intercourse; pain or ache in the testes, penis and/or rectum; urinary frequency and burning pains on passing water. Chills and fever are more likely with bacterial infection. The non-bacterial form is by far the commonest of the three and there is some indication that it can be aggravated by certain forms of exercise – jogging, squash and the like – on a full bladder. A good idea is to pee before you play. If you think you may have any of these, quit intercourse – you could pass an infection on to your partner – and go to see your doctor.

Prostate cancer will always be your main worry if you develop any of the above symptoms. Go to see the doctor and take heart, because in 99+ per cent of cases it won't be cancer, and even if it is it can usually be cured if caught in its early stages. Unfortunately, only 15 per cent of treatable prostate cancers are picked up at an early stage in the UK compared with 50 per cent in the USA, where annual screening is available. In contrast, when it comes to natural prostate treatment Europe leads the way.

YOHIMBE
Pausinystalia yohimbe
AFRICA

Yohimbe is a tree that grows throughout the forests of central and West Africa. Its flowers have conspicuous appendages reminiscent of men's genitalia, so if you believe in the Doctrine of Signatures (see p. 59) you will not find it surprising that it could be nature's answer to Viagra. Yohimbe has a long-standing reputation as an aphrodisiac and is taken internally for impotence and frigidity. Its effects include increased libido, sensation and stamina. Women and men report similar results and general pleasant sensations. Yohimbe has been used in combination with ginseng and saw palmetto (see p. 260) as a remedy for men with low sex drive. Because of its energizing influence on the endocrine system, it is widely used by athletes.

A cardiostimulant, yohimbe's energising effects stem from its ability to increase heart rate, blood pressure and hence blood flow to the genitalia. It is thought to stimulate the pelvic nerve ganglia and is thus helpful for men with erectile problems. The bark stimulates chemical reactions in the body that may help in cases of impotence caused by fatigue, tension or stress. Yohimbe reduces the effect of hormones that cause the constriction of blood vessels, which typically increases with age. It increases the production of the chemical norepinephrine, essential to the process of erection, and may boost the adrenaline supply to nerve endings, which can quicken sensual stimulation.

Yohimbine hydrochloride is the only FDA-approved drug for impotence available on prescription besides Viagra, and costs ten times more than yohimbe, which is available under brand names such as Yocon and Aphrodyne.

As with many orthodox drugs, yohimbe should only be taken under medical supervision. Subject to legal restrictions in some countries, it should not be taken by those suffering from renal or hepatic disease or using tricyclic antidepressants, which may increase the risk of hypertension.

DAMIANA
Turnera diffusa var. aphrodisiaca
CENTRAL AND SOUTH AMERICA

Now popular worldwide, Damiana has been used as an aphrodisiac since ancient times by the native people of Mexico. Traditionally, the herb is Mexico's version of Viagra and consumed only by men, although Mexican women have used it for stomach ailments, hormonal imbalance and menstrual problems. A delicious liqueur called Crème de Damiana manufactured in Guadalajara is often a visitor's first introduction to the herb.

In European herbal medicine damiana is chiefly seen as an aphrodisiac, a tonic, a promoter of digestion and an antidepressant. It has been suggested that its alkaloidal content could have a testosterone-type action that affects sexual appetite and function. This characteristic of the herb also appears to be helpful in treating premature ejaculation as well as impotence, dysmenorrhoea and menstrual headache. Recent Hawaiian research of the proprietary drug ArginMax, containing damiana, showed apparent improvement in sexual desire in women in, clitoral sensation, frequency of sexual intercourse and orgasm, and reduced vaginal dryness.

Damiana has also been used to treat urinary infections such as cystitis and urethritis, since it is both an antiseptic and a glycosidal diuretic. It is strongly antimicrobial and antiseptic, and where there is poor bowel-muscle motion the flavonoids in it act as a mild purgative.

Of the sparse research done to date, the focus has been mainly on the herb's essential oil content, which includes fragrant substances called 'terpenes'. The leaves, which have also been used as a tea substitute, contain arbutin (the antimicrobial element), alkaloids and other potentially important compounds. Indeed, not all damiana's leaf compounds are known and it is probable that the beta-sitosterol constituent also contributes towards its stimulatory effect on the sexual organs. It has recently been found that, combined with the herbs yerba maté and guarana, damiana can help to induce weight loss.

CACAO
Theobroma cacao
CENTRAL AMERICA

It will come as no surprise to many that chocolate has long been used as an aphrodisiac; the Aztecs drank *cocahutal* – cold chocolate with chilli. This was the original chocolate drink, used to maintain health and strength and stimulate sexual appetite. Early reports on the native peoples also tell us that the major pharmaceutical use of cacao was as a base for other medicines and that it was used to treat burns, bowel dysfunction, cuts and skin irritations amongst other complaints. Christopher Columbus first brought reports of cocoa to Spain from Mexico in 1502. Since then, 'hot chocolate' has been lauded by every good exponent of the sexual act, from Casanova to Madame de Pompadour.

It is now known that one constituent of chocolate, phenolethylamine (PEA), can affect our mood. PEA is a chemical similar to an amphetamine that researchers believe our body releases when we are in love. Its amphetamine-like nature is responsible for mood swings and, as with amphetamines, PEA may cause an initial lift in mood followed by a crash. Other research shows that it can help lift depression in 60 per cent of affected patients. The formula of PEA is also closely related to rosewater, produced by distilling roses, so some feel that chocolate's scent may have a powerful effect on the psyche. Other chemical components of chocolate such as anandamide, sugar and caffeine also contribute to chocolate's mood-altering action.

Recent research attests that dark chocolate has many general health benefits, and as well as being less detrimental to teeth than other sweets it is a good source of iron and magnesium. Its unique potent concentration of antioxidant flavonoids can help protect against infections and degenerative diseases, and may have anti-platelet and anticoagulant properties useful in the prevention of heart disease. The polyphenols, procyanidin flavonoids catechin and epicatechin may also help prevent cancer.

RYE
Secale cereale
TURKEY, ARMENIA

There is plenty of good news coming through on rye, on both the healthfood and the herbal medicine front. A 'good news' study of changing diets in Denmark carried out in 1995–2001 lists the increasing consumption of fresh fruit, vegetables and rye bread as a positive trend. As early as the tenth century rye was a staple in Ireland used in the distilling of spirits for medicines, proving that the saying 'just for medicinal purposes' has ancient roots. In the modern world, herbal medicine has found another role for this somewhat neglected cereal. An extract from the pollen called 'cernitin' (a Swedish word for the pure and natural substance derived from flower pollen), made using the cold-pressing process so as to protect the nutrients in the pollen grains, is used mainly for hyperlipidaemia (high blood fats) and benign prostatic hyperplasia (BHP). On the market for fifty years, Cernilton has been used by millions of men worldwide in the treatment of this disorder. In many countries the extract's efficacy has been officially approved and it is recommended by pharmacists and medical practitioners for its therapeutic value.

Cernitin supplies vital nutrients to the body cells, including all essential amino acids and enzymes. It improves the absorption of vitamins, minerals and trace elements from food, and helps to regulate many natural functions, in particular supporting the healthy function of the prostate. This means that cernitin can also help with problems to do with passing urine at night, which usually occur in elderly men with enlarged prostate glands. It is a common reason for those afflicted to request a prostatectomy. The pollen extract has been recognised as a lipid-lowering agent since 1983. Recent research suggests that rye bran in particular provides a source of dietary phenolic antioxidants that may help prevent atherosclerosis and coronary heart disease.

YERBA MATÉ

Ilex paraguensis syn. I. paraguariensis

SOUTH AMERICA

Beneath the rainforest canopy of South America, the Guarani people have drunk maté – 'the drink of the gods' – for many centuries. They were the first to discover the numerous health benefits it provides, including a strengthened immune system, improved digestion, reduced stress and stimulated mental processes. In 1964 the Pasteur Institute and the Paris Scientific Society became interested in this healthy source of vitamins and minerals and carried out a thorough study of its properties, concluding: 'It is difficult to find a plant in any area of the world equal to maté in nutritional value.' Nowadays, maté is practically a national drink in South America, and over 300,000 tonnes of the herb are produced annually for consumption in Brazil, Argentina, Uruguay and Paraguay. Maté-drinking has a very macho image, and it is also consumed in the USA, France and Germany

Research attributes maté's antioxidant action and its beneficial effects on the liver, as well as its bitter taste, to the leaves' high flavonoid and phenolic content. It is used for problems such as obesity, arthritis, headache, haemorrhoids, fluid retention, constipation, allergies and hay fever. It is also still used to stimulate the mind, to counteract fatigue and stress, to retard ageing and as a general tonic. Aqueous extracts of *I. paraguariensis* are more potent antioxidants than ascorbic acid (vitamin C). Other maté constituents include caffeine and saponins; vitamins B_6, C, niacin and pantothenic acid; sodium, calcium, copper, iron, zinc, potassium, especially magnesium and manganese. All that in a tea-leaf, now readily available in an unpatented tea-bag.

Yerba maté may be able to alleviate the fast-increasing Western obesity problem, endemic in both America and the UK. In 2001 a herbal remedy called Zotrim, nineteen years in the making by Dane Dr Lasse Hessel, came on to the market. It combines yerba maté with damiana (which has laxative, tonic and hormonal applications) and guarana (see p. 256). This combination has proved useful in the battle against slimmers' 'yo-yo' syndrome, for it causes and maintains weight loss by harmlessly delaying the emptying of the stomach, thereby, extending the duration of the early stages of digestion. It also makes it less attractive for users to over-indulge, as the uncomfortably full feeling lingers longer.

SAW PALMETTO
Serenoa repens
NORTH AMERICA

Saw palmetto grows along the dunes of the Atlantic coast, and in dense underbrush on Florida's eastern seaboard. Its seeds used to be eaten by the locals and their animals, reputedly making the latter sleek and fat. They also used the fruit as a diuretic and sexual tonic. The Seminole people of Florida used the fruits for food and the leaf stems for basket-making. An infusion of the berries was employed as a digestive and for dysentery. Today saw palmetto is more likely to make its appearance on the Florida Keys in Prosnut Butter, a nutty spread consumed by those suffering from benign prostate hyperplasia.

In the nineteenth century serenoa fruits and pulp were used as a tonic, and by the early twentieth the fruits were being used for prostatic conditions. Saw palmetto contains chiefly carbohydrates, and it is thought to work by reducing levels of a very active form of the male hormone testosterone known as dihydrotestosterone (DHT), considered to be the primary cause of enlargement of the prostate. In the States, research has shown a 90 per cent success rate in treating the condition with saw palmetto, which is said to be a better result than pharmaceutical drugs or surgery can boast. Serenoa herbal preparations have been reported to be twenty-five times stronger than orthodox drugs and they have none of the nasty side-effects. The herb is also used in traditional Western medicine for problems such as chronic or subacute cystitis, impotence, wasting diseases, catarrh of the genito-urinary tract and sex hormone disorders. The anabolic and tonic action strengthens and builds body tissues and encourages weight gain. Saw palmetto is also useful, when taken internally, to women for breast enlargement, and most recently in a pilot study it was found to be an effective treatment for baldness.

GINSENG
Panax ginseng

CHINA

Now rare in the wild, *Panax ginseng* is cultivated extensively in North and South Korea, China, Japan and Russia to satisfy the massive worldwide demand for this ancient Taoist herb. Ginseng's name is derived from the Doctrine of Signatures (see p. 59) and the Chinese ideogram for 'crystallisation of the essence of the earth in the form of man'. Ginseng has been an integral part of Chinese medicine for over three thousand years, a reputed panacea for cancer, rheumatism, diabetes and sexual debility; and regarded as an aphrodisiac and as effective against ageing. Today, it is an ingredient in many important Chinese herbal formulae. In the West, it is used more as a lifestyle tonic than as a medicine and is taken for lack of appetite, insomnia, stress and shock amongst other disorders, as well as for chronic illness. It can improve mental health and social functioning after about four weeks' therapy, but the benefits diminish with continued use.

In the male department, *Panax ginseng* has been shown to increase both the motility and the quantity of spermatozoa; it may be a useful agent in preventing and treating testicular damage induced by environmental pollutants. Ginseng has also been shown to be a tonic or 'adaptogen' that enhances physical performance (including sexual) and promotes vitality. Adaptogens, as described by leading Soviet scientist Dr I. I. Brekhman, help normalise body functions – for example, those relating to blood pressure and blood sugar. They appear to work best on people who are neither in ill health nor in the peak of condition; and ginseng 'brings out the best in ordinary people'. Trials show that it can significantly improve the body's capacity to cope with hunger, extremes of temperature and mental and emotional stress. These properties are believed to be due to its effects on the hypothalamic-pituitary-adrenal axis. Research since the 1980s has confirmed that *Panax ginseng* has anti-senility effects, helping to relieve many of the symptoms of ageing.

Ginseng, its saponins and ginsenosides are also likely to be instrumental in the herb's ability to modulate pain in animals 'in vivo' and 'in vitro' respectively and have potential to aid spinal cord injuries. 'Ginseng has been used for thousands of years in the treatment of neurological disorders and other diseases in Asia. Ginsenosides Rb1 and Rg1 represent potentially effective therapeutic agents for spinal cord injuries'.

Ginseng lowers anticoagulant levels and may not be taken with anticoagulant drugs such as warfarin or the antidepressant phenelzine. Recently, Korean, Russian and Chinese research on both animals and humans points to ginseng holding considerable promise for future cancer prevention; indeed, a ginseng-based anti-cancer drug has already been produced in China.

PYGEUM

Pygeum africanum.

CENTRAL AND SOUTHERN AFRICA

In Africa, the bark of the Pygeum tree is traditionally powdered and drunk as a 'tea' for genito-urinary complaints. European interest in Pygeum began as early as the 1700s, when tribal medicine men in Natal showed early settlers how the bark helped cure bladder pains. In the 1960s a French entrepreneur, Debat, lodged the first patent for Pygeum bark extract to treat prostate disorders. Soon the fat-soluble extract of Pygeum bark became the primary treatment for an enlarged prostate gland in France. The success of this treatment (which fuelled a US $220 million annual market) put the tree in jeopardy of extinction and caused severe shortages – prompting action to conserve the wild tree species in Africa.

Today Pygeum bark extract is used for enlargement of the prostate or Benign Prostatic Hyperplasia (BPH). This is believed to be caused by an extremely active form of testosterone (dihydroxytestosterone [DHT]). Widespread tests show that Pygeum treatment significantly reduces prostate size and clears obstructions of the bladder neck and urethra. In comparison, synthetic drugs and surgery – the two normal options for BPH – can cause some serious side effects, including impotence and incontinence.

Pygeum bark contains three groups of active constituents that combat the effects of BPH: phyto-sterols that have anti-inflammatory effects; Pentacyclic triterpenoids that have a decongesting action and ferulic esters that reduce levels of the hormone prolactin (which stimulates and maintains the secretion of milk) and block the accumulation of cholesterol in the prostate. The later effect is of special significance because prolactin increases uptake of testosterone by the prostate, and cholesterol increases binding sites for DHT. The majority of the studies report an absence of any significant adverse effects of Pygeum, although there have been rare complaints of diarrhoea, constipation, dizziness, gastric pain, and visual disturbances. Although pygeum has been the subject of some controversy, mainly in reviews of past research rather than more investment and active interest in doing the level of research required by the medical and pharmaceutical establishments, in conclusion, pygeum extracts certainly appear to have some efficacy in ameliorating symptoms of lower urinary tract symptoms (LUTS) and mild to modest BPH.

18

A Woman's World

The *mons Veneris*, 'mountain of love', is a shapely curve of fatty tissue, hidden and protected beneath which is the flexible joint between the right and left pubic bones that ease open during childbirth. Below this shock-absorber are two long folds of skin flanking the entrance of the vagina, which is well supplied with oil and sweat glands.

The clitoris This is a cylindrical bundle of eight thousand nerve fibres and fully formed at twenty-seven weeks after conception, it will grow to a length of about 16 millimetres. Like its male counterpart, the penis, when stimulated it can become softly erect. It does so not by clamping the venous outflow but by speeding arterial inflow, and erection and orgasm can therefore be multiple. Like all good sensory organs the clitoris can be a harbinger of pleasure or of sorrow (the latter in those countries that still practise clitoral circumcision).

The urethra It has only one job to do, and that is to transport the urine out of the body – no added complication of having act to as an exit route for other products of the loins.

The vagina This tunnel, 10–13 centimetres long, has amazing potential for accommodating penises or just-about-to-be-born babies; and just as it can open, it can also close and grip. The vagina is home to legions of bacteria, which *should* be there. They are goodies, producing acidic organic bactericides that can stop the baddies in their tracks. A healthy vagina is as clean and as pure as a pot of organic yoghurt, and so it should remain throughout life.

The cervix Shaped like a doughnut, the cervix is the mouth of the uterus and can open to let the menstrual fluid escape, or shut tight to hold the baby inside the womb for the regulation nine months.

The uterus At rest, the uterus is only about 8 centimetres long and weighs around 60 grams, but during pregnancy it expands a thousand-fold. This, the original solar-powered intensive-care unit, is mainly made of muscle; it is capable not only of responding to the internal web of hormonal messaging, but is more than capable of putting its own chemical spoke in when necessary, which prompts the smooth muscle to contract.

The oviducts These two pencil-thin tubes are topped by a crest of tiny pink fingers. Each finger moves, caressing the surface of the ovary it appears to serve. However, as the need arises, each can waft its atten-tion in the other ovary's direction. Each is a mobile stethoscope seek-ing information as to where the egg will erupt in its moment of free-dom in the body cavity. Then the ordered ranks of beating cilia that line the gentle fingers take charge, cupping and then cajoling the egg down into the confines of the nuptial chamber first described in the sixteenth century by one Gabriel Fallopius. The walls of the fallopian tubes now undergo peristalsis, gently helping the egg along on its three-day journey. Unless it is fertilised the egg can only live for only about twenty-four hours, so perhaps it is only the fittest sperm that reaches its goal, high up in one of the tubes. Using the magic of mini-cameras strapped to willing penises, scientific paparazzi have obtained evidence that part of the female orgasm includes the cervix reaching down into the uterus to help the sperm on their way.

The happy union accomplished, the two sets of genes mix and a unique embryo results. Yes, each one of us is unique – so unique that the uterus wall must be specially prepared in order to receive the alien ball of cells.

One of my first lectures to biology undergraduates attempted to define the difference between an organic being, a living organism and dead, non-organic raw material. All living things move, however slow-ly; are irritable – that is, they respond to often minute stimuli; grow and develop; respire; and reproduce. And they use an energy source to do all these things. So am I alive? The answer is no, not in the complete fulfilment of the definition, for neither my wife nor I can reproduce on our own. In the case of *Homo sapiens* and the vast majority of other animals and plants, the complete fulfilment of the definition of life is a team of two. Neither is completely in the driving seat.

If you are tempted to say I am being pedantic, that he or she has the potential for reproducing, so he or she is alive, how about all those trace elements they have? Thanks to Creation, evolution, creative evolution or whatever you like to call it, they too have the potential to be part of a living package, but they don't have the potential to reproduce themselves. Also, unless the environment and our energy supply are just right, then we are, in biological terms, a dead end. Matter can neither be created nor destroyed, life is the only thing that can create more of itself, and life is the only thing that can die. Perhaps the poet Samuel Butler hit it on the head when he said that life 'is the art of drawing sufficient conclusions from insufficient premises'.

Halfway through her life as a foetus, safe inside her mum, every woman-to-be has some six to seven million eggs already held in her two embryonic ovaries. Four million of these will self-destruct in the next twenty weeks, and by puberty only four hundred thousand will remain. Of these no more than 450 will be released ready for fertilisation, and at the menopause few if any will be left. Her body will have reclaimed all but those lucky enough to be turned into an embryo and breathe fresh air.

Each month, throughout the fertile life of a female of the species one egg, and in very rare cases more, will be released into the body cavity. The egg then makes its way slowly along the oviduct, during which time it must meet the right sperm if fertilisation is to occur. Even before the egg erupts from the follicle in the ovary, the wall of the uterus has undergone changes ready to receive the fertile egg. The empty follicle does not go to waste, but changes into the corpus luteum, whose job it is to secrete the hormone progesterone that helps speed maturation of the uterine wall ready for implantation. This process takes about three days. If all these things don't come together, then implantation is impossible. The corpus luteum degenerates, slowing the flow of progesterone to the uterine wall, which is sloughed off, and the blood and debris are passed out as the menstrual flow.

If the hormones of the dad- and mum-to-be do get it all together, a foetus will result and another human being is on the way. If all its cells have two X chromosomes and there is just enough oestrogen about it will be a girl, already complete with another six or seven million eggs. Like her mum and dad she will be endowed with some reproductive traits that are not found in the rest of the animal kingdom.

Despite the fact that we don't do it in public, which as David Attenborough has proved most other sorts of animals do, we have sex repeatedly – even when the female of the species is not ovulating and there is no hope of a conception – which most other animals don't do. Another unique attribute of our sex life revolves around the fact that the females, and in very rare cases the male, undergo peoplopause (don't go looking in the dictionary for that one). In effect they become sterile, and yet they continue to enjoy having sex for the rest of their lives. Other mammals would never do such a thing, although as they remain fertile to death does them part, they don't have the problem.

Until they are three or four years old, the bloodstreams of both sexes receive minute pulses of reproductive hormone, one about every ninety minutes. These are secreted by a special structure in the hypothalamus. During this time both sexes become slightly erotic about their bodies, especially the rude bits that begin to fascinate them. Then for the next six years or so the little pre-sex stopcock stops dripping. At some point the adrenals mature, kindling the flames of sexuality, and about two years later the sex stopcock deep in the brain is turned on again. From this point the ovaries or the testes take over as the primary source of the sex drive.

Four weeks into their life both male and female foetuses, like all other mammals, have milk ridges extending from their armpits to their groins. In the evolutionary cause of waste-not-want-not, and what with the peculiarities of bipedalism and the upright stance, minimum litter size and cuddle-suckling, only the top two potential mammae develop; and then only when stimulated by enough of the right hormone. Human females differ from all their closest relatives in developing large breasts from the start. The rest have nipples, but don't grow large boobs until they need them to feed their young. What is more, mums with small breasts produce just as much milk as those with big ones. So there has been over the years no selective advantage in a male finding beauty in the breast and choosing a big-breasted mate, for their offspring will not get a bigger ration of milk.

Please remember that in biological terms the main function of the male and female of any species is to produce a vehicle that will set the whole thing in motion again and carry their genes on to infinity and beyond. That is the essence of survival. So it is not surprising that recent research indicates that in young girls it is body weight, and especially plumpness, that speeds sexual maturity. Plump girls tend to menstruate earlier than thin or athletic girls, the explanation being that when the body has saved up enough energy to run the intensive care unit, all systems are ready for up and go.

And don't forget the importance of good food during pregnancy: special enriched diets are of course recommended for mums-to-be. And would-be dads too, why not join the club and get prepared for all those broken nights and nappies? A word of advice: never make light of those food fads – lobster, strawberries, oysters, green vegetables, avocado and the like. All are good natural sources of those special omega-6 and omega-3 unsaturated (brain-building) fatty acids and/or trace elements. Mum always does know best – and get ready for a Madame Curie or Albert Einstein in the family.

It is a truism to say that a breast-fed baby could not be better fed, for the flow of mother's milk is one of the wonders of creative evolution. First, the fat-free yellow colostrum full of the building-blocks of vitamins A and B, white blood cells and antibodies: mother's own baby formula produced on demand to bolster the baby's immune system, which is still far from mature. Then the pure white milk, nature's perfect food, very sweet thanks to lactose, a sugar that not only contains twice as much energy as glucose but ensures the conservation of calcium and other raw materials essential to growth. To push the point well and truly home, an Australian study of sixteen hundred babies that had died in accidents or from non-heart-related problems found early damage to blood vessels, and this was seven times more prevalent in bottle- than in breast-fed babies.

Research has also shown that the gradual introduction of gluten-containing foods into the diet of infants while they are still being breast-fed reduces the risk of coeliac disease in early childhood, and probably also during later childhood. So changes of diet should be taken seriously and undertaken with care.

BLACK COHOSH
Cimicifuga racemosa syn. Actaea
NORTH AMERICA

Black cohosh has an extensive history of use by Native Americans, who revered it as a remedy for a host of common ailments. The root acquired the names 'black snakeroot' from its reputation as an antidote to the bite of the rattlesnake, and 'squawroot' from its association with female problems. Although now known worldwide as a remedy for women's cyclical conditions, it is an 'all ages' family herb that was used for problems common to both sexes such as fatigue, kidney ailments and respiratory infections; it was also considered beneficial for children with whooping cough and, as a syrup, in cases of St Vitus' dance. Adopted from the Native Americans by New World settlers, black cohosh was used by them and their herbal doctors. In the 1840s the Eclectic physicians used it for many manifestations of illness, particularly rheumatic pain.

Black cohosh products are now regularly used in Europe for the treatment of PMS, period pains, other menstrual problems and the menopause. It is now the largest-selling herbal dietary supplement in the USA for alleviating symptoms associated with the menopause.

Black cohosh influences the endocrine regulatory system, with effects similar to one of the milder endogenous oestrogens, oestriol. The herb's oestrogen-like action is thought to be responsible for decreasing the ovaries' production of progesterone. In 1995 black cohosh combined with St John's wort was found to be 78 per cent successful at treating hot flushes and other menopausal problems; it may be that the oestrogen-like action of black cohosh may depend here on its being part of a compound. Recent American research has found extracts to be useful for younger women suffering hormonal deficits following the removal of ovaries or uterus, as well as for juvenile disorders. Consult a healthcare professional before using the extracts for hormonal purposes, or if you have liver problems.

SWEET HONEYLEAF
Stevia rebaudiana

The usefulness of sweet honeyleaf (*caä-éhé*, or 'sweet herb') was first discovered by the Guarani people of Paraguay over fifteen hundred years ago, long before the arrival of Columbus. It was brought to the attention of Europeans only in the 1880s, and not until a hundred years later was it developed as the sweetener and flavour-enhancer that is now used widely in many countries. Today in America, growing a plant in a pot or window-box as a no-calorie herbal sugar substitute has become a popular pastime. It is estimated that 30 millilitres of *Stevia* extract is equivalent to 3 kilograms of sucrose. *Stevia* in its natural herb form is approximately ten to fifteen times sweeter than common table sugar. It also has a useful nutritive value and is a good source of vitamin C, beta-carotene and minerals. Traditionally the herb has been used as a cardiotonic, as an antiflatulent and for obesity, as well as to reduce heartburn, hypertension and uric acid levels. Science has recently confirmed that it has a hypotensive effect in animals.

Studies suggest that sweet honeyleaf has a regulating effect on the pancreas and could help stabilise blood-sugar levels in the body, making it useful for diabetes, hypoglycaemia and candidiasis (thrush). Research also validates its antibacterial use. It is non-toxic, does not adversely affect blood sugar, and inhibits the formation of cavities and plaque. The Japanese have been using it for thirty years in confectionery and bakery. Its sweetner component has advantages over artificial sweeteners, as it is stable at high temperatures (100°C), has a pH range of 3–9, and does not darken with cooking. In South America it is used in such products as soft drinks, ice-cream, biscuits, pickles, chewing-gum, tea and skin preparations. At a time when in the West obesity with all its disease-related complications is a fast-growing concern, sweet honeyleaf could offer a potentially groundbreaking role as an alternative healthy substitute for sugar.

The plant's pollen can be highly allergenic to certain individuals.

COTTON
Gossypium spp.

Recent archaeological research on the gulf coast of Tabasco, Mexico, has found that domesticated cotton appeared as farming expanded c. 2500 BC, but it is said that the Maya and Aztecs were using the pollen medicinally as early as 3400 BC. It was being cultivated in Asia in 2500 BC, and introduced as a herb from India to Egypt and China around 500 BC.

America's first people used the root bark to ease childbirth pains and as lint for mopping up other problems. In Europe and the UK, cotton root's main use was as a labour-inducing herb and for menstrual problems such as heavy bleeding, and it was used to help clot blood and to encourage the secretion of breast-milk. Cotton seed is used to treat endometriosis (the presence of tissue similar to the lining of the uterus at other sites in the pelvis, such as the ovaries, fallopian tubes and pelvic ligaments). The root of *G. hirsutum* was commonly used as an abortefacient, shutting down the corpus luteum's ability to produce progesterone, essential to the continuation of pregnancy. In Western herbalism, Levant cotton (*G. herbaceum*) root bark is used to stimulate uterine contractions, and can alleviate amenorrhoea and painful menstruation as caused, for instance, by obstructions such as fibroids.

Containing the anti-fertility compound gossypol, cotton seed oil lowers sperm production, and in 2000 Chinese research pointed to it having a contraceptive effect in men. In 2002, research indicated its possible use as a contraceptive drug for men. Cotton seeds have been used for dysentery and fever, and externally for skin viruses and irritations, lacerations and lesions, as well as inflammation of the testes. The leaves have been taken for inflammation of the stomach and intestines and used externally for candidiasis, ulceration, water-vapour burns and contusions.

In a practical everyday sense, pure cotton T-shirts offer some protection against UV radiation, essential for adults and children alike when holidaying in sunnier climes. There is only one real problem with this plant: its cultivation necessitates the use of lots of agricultural chemicals and an inordinate amount of irrigation (a main factor in creating salt deserts across the arid world and of the demise of the Aral Sea).

Cotton root bark and cotton seed oil are for use only under the supervision of qualified practitioners. Do not use during pregnancy.

RASPBERRY
Rubus idaeus
EUROPE, ASIA, NORTH AMERICA

The raspberry fruit was first mentioned in Chinese medical literature c. 500 AD and the plant was one of the most important for the *Carrier*, a group of native people of north-central British Columbia who passed their knowledge on to the European settlers in the nineteenth century. Now eaten mainly as a soft summer fruit, it is known to be highly nutritive and to contain antioxidants and anticarcinogenic anthocyanins.

Raspberry leaves have long been connected with female health, including pregnancy. Leaf tea was considered a remedy for excessive menstrual flow and was used in pregnancy to help prevent complications. It was thought to tone the tissue of the womb, assisting contractions by strengthening its longitudinal muscle, and to check any haemorrhaging during labour. Raspberry leaves are used in traditional medicines as an astringent for diarrhoea, leucorrhoea (an abnormal vaginal discharge) and other conditions such as mouth problems, and as a gargle for sore throats. The plant has also been used for morning sickness, diabetes, bronchitis and coughs. Raspberry-tops tea is used to relieve symptoms of colds and flu, acute respiratory inflammation and erysipelas (an inflammatory skin disease).

In 1999 raspberry leaf and its effect on labour – especially its safety and efficacy – were investigated in a retrospective study comprising 108 mothers, just over half of whom had been using raspberry leaf while pregnant. It was found that ingestion of the drug might have decreased the likelihood of gestation problems.

Also, the mothers who had used it were less likely to have their membranes ruptured, or to require a Caesarean section or a forceps or vacuum birth. More recent Australian research into the safety and efficacy of raspberry-leaf tablets used in labour has suggested that it is safe for both mother and baby, that it shortens the second stage of labour and offers a reduction in the use of forceps deliveries of over 10 per cent.

Excessive use of raspberry can cause mild loosening of stools and nausea, and it interacts with certain prescribed drugs including codeine. It may not be taken in the first trimester of pregnancy.

CHASTEBERRY
Vitex agnus-castus
ITALY, GREECE, MEDITERRANEAN

The chasteberry's peppery fruits have been used medicinally for at least two millennia. A traditional white-flowered chastity symbol, the plant has been used to treat constipation, flatulence, hangovers and fevers. It was early recognised for its ability to bring on menstruation and to relieve uterine cramps. Nineteenth-century American Eclectic physicians used it to induce menstrual flow and to stimulate lactation in nursing women.

Chasteberry has always been considered an important herb for regulating female hormones, and it is still used for that purpose. It is used in Western herbal medicine to treat menstrual irregularities such as pre-menstrual syndrome (PMS), including the breast tenderness that may accompany it. It is also used to encourage fertility and breast-milk production. However, officially the herb is not recommended for use during pregnancy or lactation, and you should also be aware of any interactions with other herbs or drugs that might contraindicate its use.

GINGER ROOT
Zingiber officinale
ASIA

Ginger was recorded in early Sanskrit and Chinese texts and in ancient Greek, Roman and Arabic medical literature. Traditional Chinese and Asian medical practitioners have used dried ginger, *gan jiang*, as a remedy for 'internal cold', and it is used to treat problems such as abdominal pain, lumbago and diarrhoea. Fresh ginger, *shen jiang*, which is also a culinary herb, is used for vomiting, coughs, abdominal distension and fever. In Africa ginger root is similarly used, and in the Ayurvedic pharmacopoeia the plant is called *vishwabhesaj*, 'the universal medicine', and employed as a digestive and respiratory herb. In the West, ginger is considered anti-inflammatory, antiseptic, anti-emetic and carminative, and it is also used as a circulatory stimulant and an antussive (to inhibit coughing).

Ginger is well researched for its therapeutic benefits, which are chiefly due to its volatile oil and resin. Although not formally recognised for motion and morning sickness in the USA, the UK employs ginger for its traditional ability to counter digestive complaints such as indigestion, nausea, wind and colic, but also to relieve travel sickness and morning sickness in pregnancy. Research has shown that ginger's components gingerol and shogaol suppress gastric contractions, and a study of capsules containing the dried rhizome found them to be superior to an antihistamine in preventing the gastrointestinal symptoms of motion sickness. In 1990, trials in England found the herb more effective than conventional medicines in relieving post-operative nausea (particularly useful in day-case surgery).

Recent research indicates that shogaols extracted from ginger may hold good neurological news for the unborn and the aged.

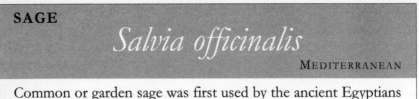

SAGE
Salvia officinalis
MEDITERRANEAN

Common or garden sage was first used by the ancient Egyptians as a remedy for infertility. The Greek physician Dioscorides declared that it stopped bleeding and cleansed wounds and sores, while Pliny the Elder found sage enhanced memory function and prescribed it for mouth and throat problems. This aromatic, astringent herb has been used by all the herbal disciplines world-wide.

Sage continues to be used in traditional Western herbal medicine as a gargle or mouthwash for pharyngitis, tonsillitis and similar disorders. Used as a culinary herb, it has been said to cut fat and aid digestion. It is also useful for mild diarrhoea and as an infusion to reduce perspiration, and may be found in modern antiperspirants. In Ayurvedic medicine sage is used to promote hair growth, and is said to have a special power to clear emotional obstructions and render the mind calm and clear.

Today the herb is a valued remedy for menstrual problems, such as irregular periods or amenorrhoea. Its leaf oil contains a mild amount of thujone which, although toxic in excess, has been proved to be a powerful antiseptic and to give warming relief for digestive disorders. Thujone also has an oestrogenic action, which medical herbalists describe as aiding the muscles of the uterus during childbirth. Sage is used to alleviate menopausal symptoms such as the hot flushes and insomnia inducing nocturnal sweats that reflect the body's adaptation to oestrogen deprivation.

Epileptics should not use thujone-containing herbs. Sage also decreases lactation and should therefore be avoided during pregnancy and breast-feeding.

WILD YAM, MEXICAN YAM
Dioscorea spp.

It was only in the 1950s that a brilliant young biochemist, Russell E. Marker, made a herbal discovery that perhaps more than any other has changed the world. He found that the wild yam produces human sex hormones – or rather, that its constituent diosgesin can, with the flick of the biochemist's test tube, be turned into the female hormone progesterone and then easily transformed into testosterone. It was because of this property that it became the basis of the female contraceptive pill. Despite the fact that this happened back in the years of Flower Power, both the scientific world and the company for which Marker worked were incredulous of his claims. So he packed his bags and set off to Mexico where he set up his own company, Syntex, which produced the oral contraceptive pill. The rest is herbal history, for it not only revolutionised sex but gave the world a real chance to plan the size of its future family. Then, of course along came the spectre of AIDS, which brought condoms and another sort of plant (the Hevea brasiliensis, rubber) back into the picture. It is also forgotten that the progesterone produced from the Mexican yam played its part in the making of another miracle drug, cortisone.

Marker was not, however, the first to use the yam. Tradition has it that the root of the wild Mexican yam was used medicinally by the Maya and Aztec people of South America. Centuries later, other Native Americans and then the settlers used the twisting rhizome of the perennial vine to treat menstrual, ovarian and labour pains and other gynaecological problems, as well such ailments as rheumatism and arthritis. *Shan yao* (*D. batatas*) has been used in Chinese folkloric and traditional medicine for over two thousand years as a body, mind and spirit herb to counteract the emotional instability associated with *qi* (physical 'life-force') deficiency, which in women may be attributed to the menopause and traditionally indicates hormonal influence. In Ayurvedic medicine, wild yam species are considered to have sweet, bitter, cooling energies and were variously employed for impotence, senility, hormonal deficiency, infertility and other problems. The American yam, too, is considered an effective tonic for the female reproductive system and is also used for bronchitis, catarrh, asthma, whooping cough and cramp, and as a homoeopathic remedy for colic, especially in infants.

Research has shown that wild yam contains alkaloids and other saponins, some of which have exhibited promising cardiovascular and anti-tumour action. In-vitro studies show that wild yam root is anti-oestrogenic. While diosgenin, as Marker demonstrated in the 1950s, can certainly be used in the laboratory as a source of sex hormones, it cannot be converted in the body into progesterone or other sex hormones.

RED CLOVER
Trifolium pratense
EUROPE, AND ASIA

Wild Red Clover is a familiar plant native to Europe, North Africa and Central Asia, which down the ages has been of good service in many ways. In medieval times it provided the most important leguminous forage crop in northern Europe. Today, scientists know that clover offers cattle a rich source of Vitamins A and E and that the fixed nitrogen in the nodules on its roots is in effect free fertiliser. Children still love hunting in a patch of red clover for a rare four-leafed specimen, which is kept to bring 'good luck', and it is the blossoms of this species that are employed in herbalism. Red clover is used in many blends of herbal extracts and capsules to nourish the body's ability to cleanse and enhance the liver and intestinal tract functions. It also helps the body to produce healthy blood cells that are essential to the maintenance of all organs and systems. Current interest in Red clover's flowers focuses on their use to relieve menopausal symptoms, and recent research suggests that the plant's isoflavone compound genistein could be potentially useful in the treatment of those symptoms.

Plants produce over 1000 different isoflavones, water-soluble chemicals that act like estrogens, of these formononetin, daidzein, biochanin, and genistein show the greatest activity and some herbal Red clover products contain all 4. There is some controversy regarding Red clover research but promising results are being reported all the time. A trial of menopausal women taking red clover isoflavone for 16 weeks found a 50% reduction in hot flush incidence and 47% reduction in severity of hot flushes. A Dutch study on a Red Clover remedy Promensil, (Novogen Ltd., Australia) reported a 16% and 44% reduction in hot flushes in post-menopausal women within one and two months respectively. Some studies suggest that a proprietary extract of red clover isoflavones may slow bone loss and even boost bone mineral density in pre- and perimenopausal women. Perhaps, in the future, for people who are on anti-coagulant medication such as aspirin it may be possible with monitoring to substitute red clover tea or tincture, or to reduce the amount of anti-coagulant drug required. Women with a history of breast cancer or those recieving hormone therapy (including birth control pills) containing estrogen, progesterone, androgen or any derivatives should avoid red clover. Also because of the increased risk of bleeding associated with red clover, individuals taking blood-thinning medications (such as warfarin or aspirin) or blood-thinning herbs and supplements (such as ginkgo, ginger, garlic, and vitamin E) should avoid red clover and only use it under medical supervision. Red clover is a classic example of a simple plant with a complex of health assistance to offer that really does require more attention and research.

19

The Patter of Little Feet

There is increasing evidence that, despite the wonders of mother's milk, malnutrition of mums both before and during pregnancy and suckling can have disastrous effects on a number of aspects of the development and health of their children. The differences in the genetic inheritance of the different socio economic groups cannot be entirely to blame for this. The fact that, despite our family planning clinics and health education programmes, Britain leads the world in unwanted teenage pregnancies is a factor that cannot be ignored. Likewise – or perhaps I should say 'likestupid' – the current epidemic of smoking, especially in young mothers-to-be, is frightening indeed. We now know that tobacco, like many other drugs, can take its toll on the well-being of the foetus. Danish researchers have found signs of atherosclerosis in the umbilical arteries of mothers who smoke. In puzzling contrast, despite the fast pace of life in their overcrowded cities polluted by industry and transport and the fact that they smoke the equivalent of six thousand cigarettes per person per year, the Japanese have low rates of cancer of the lung, breast and colon and of heart disease. There is evidence to show that the Japanese diet helps protect them from these Western ills. Japanese fishing fleets scour the world's oceans to help keep them supplied with the fruits of the sea.

What is more – and to digress, though I make no apology for doing so – the Japanese are the driving force behind a resumption of the harvesting (although knowing what we now know about whales and dolphins, I would call it the *murder*) of the cetaceans. They argue that the body parts of these, the most sentient of wild creatures, are part of their ethnic diet, and there is no getting away from the fact that their diet has served them well across time, especially when it comes to first-class supplies of brain food (see p. 000). The fact is that they only started to dine *extensively* on the body parts of these cetaceans in the awful wake of commercial whaling – a trade that supplied the West with nothing more important than oil for use in animal feed, margarine, soaps, and cosmetics, bone for debilitating corsets and, of course, short-term profit.

As I write this chapter there are reports in the papers warning that gross over-fishing of the world's oceans is sending more and more commercial species to the wall of extinction. Also, that the fish being caught in the fishing grounds around industrialised countries, and those farmed by intensive Western methods, are carrying an ever greater load of toxic and cancer-producing pollutants. The future looks bleak for our biochemistry unless something is done radically – and soon – to change the way we feed ourselves. And as a grandfather who has had the privilege to help raise five children, four of them adopted from different ethnic gene stock, and as a patron of the Hyperactive Children's Support Group in Britain, I must express concern for the complexity of all our futures.

I include the following extract from Janet Aiken's *The Bionutritional Basis of Mental Illness: A New Approach to Understanding and Treatment*, which has certainly put things into a better perspective for me. Though the focus here is on mental illness, the implications for every other aspect of our lives are clear:

> The search for a solution to the problem of mental illness is not to look for yet another drug to mask the symptoms, but to find out what has gone wrong with the brain's chemistry that is making it malfunction. Despite extensive investigations of genetic causes, there is no evidence that anyone is born mentally ill. There is more likely a predisposition or susceptibility to specific kinds of nervous system malfunctioning, which is aggravated by inappropriate or inadequate nutrition in conjunction with severe or chronic emotional stress:
>
> The brain and nervous system require at least 40 different nutrients to develop and function properly. If any one of these is depleted, excessive or inactivated, some psychological function will be affected. These nutrients are needed as catalysts or enzymes, regulators and raw materials for the synthesis of brain and nervous system structures and neurotransmitters. They are provided by the diet only if it is adequate and appropriate to the

individual. They can be substantially depleted, by stressors of many kinds.

Food sensitivities almost always accompany more commonly recognized environmental allergies, such as to pollen, fur, feathers, dust, moulds, etc. The adrenal glands activate the immune system to fight the foreign proteins, deal with the allergens and also cope with the emotional stress. When a person's diet routinely, and for long periods, contains foods to which the individual is sensitive, the adrenals can become run down. This would be similar to an automobile's battery running down when the headlights are left on overnight.

When major emotional stress occurs, the adrenals may not be able to respond adequately and a psychotic episode can ensue . . . Adrenal function is also severely impaired when the adrenals are overworked by exposure to food and environmental sensitivities.

The brain has preferential needs for specific vitamins, minerals, amino acids and essential fatty acids in order to function normally. Nutritional technology has advanced to the point where an individual's nutritional status in terms of specific nutrients can be identified for therapeutic nutritional intervention. Heavy metal toxicity can be identified and eliminated. Offending foods can be removed from the diet. A stable serum glucose level can be achieved. It certainly should be the policy of those professionals working with the mentally ill to address bionutritional problems, putting nutritionists (not dietitians, who are untrained in this kind of work) into every facility where mental illness is being treated. Studies have shown that nutritional intervention increases the patients' response to therapy and can often return them to normal functioning where other approaches without nutritional therapy have failed. We must all pray that such a system of nutritional screening will be put into place as rapidly as possible.

And until this happens, the family and – dare I say it in these modern days? – the extended family unit will continue to be of great importance. We need the combined wisdom of the family, the older members with their knowledge of food and illness problems and of the nutritional and medicinal successes of the past, and the younger ones who can help their elders to be cool in a rapidly changing society and with their twenty-first-century expertise surf the web for organic food news, and more.

The image of the world as a global village has never been more apposite. The weekly shopping expedition is now a grand-tour experience, with packets and labels showing us that our daily bread and all the things that go with it are now grown around the world for our convenience.

Family meals, starting with breakfast, are a time to test things out, both good and bad. 'Wow! A real cool taste!' and similar spontaneous expressions of appreciation can make the meal and bond the family, perhaps better than the rather formal graces of my youth. In like manner, rejection of a familiar food or some strange nuance of behaviour could be a warning of a genetic difference that will allow some substance to trigger hyperactivity or other antisocial behaviour. This is where the doctor-within-the-family-circle notion comes in – an essential part of the fitness of *Homo sapiens* for at least half a million years. Perhaps health wisdom really is the sixth sense.

Bathtime has always been a family affair, at least until the stirrings of puberty raise their blushing heads. Did you know that when you were inside your mum you were in a private bath, your own intensive care unit? (How did you get out? Well, that's a long story.) Home confinements may have had their problems, but they did teach all the family a lot. The modern attitude in good hospitals and health centres is great, for a new baby can still be the most important part of the family affair there. The most important thing the midwife did for you was to slap your bottom and start you breathing.

Then there's the bedtime story, one of the greatest aids to literacy and a time of sharing and real bonding. In many families prayers are as natural as the night, which could be full of fear without them. And the importance of those other shared moments, when everyone vies for a place in the family bed, should not be forgotten. There can be no better bonding experience than being part of a Mummy-and-Daddy sandwich, with a little cuddling arm in between.

Death, especially in the family, is of course a sad time, for years made ever harder to handle by the grim churchyard and even grimmer crematorium. The new preference for woodland burials, in which the passing of a loved one results in the birth of a tree, holds out the promise of some kind of continuity and of a new nearness to Mother Earth.

WILD ROSE, DOG ROSE
Rosa canina

TEMPERATE EUROPE, ASIA

'Unkempt about those hedgerows grows the unofficial English rose', a beloved emblem of all that England stood for, and of great importance in the heritage of herbal healing. Wild rosehips contain, weight for weight, as much antioxidant vitamin C as oranges. Rosehip syrup helped sustain Britain's babies during the Second World War, and is still a nutritive thirst-quenching summer drink for babies and infants. Egyptians, Persians, Greeks and Romans in classical times used the rose as a garden ornament and for various perfumes and cosmetics. Rosehip is considered a sour herb in Ayurvedic medicine and is used as an astringent, carminative and stimulant.

Today it is used as a diuretic and a tonic. Rosehip's tannins offer a gentle aid to gastric upset and diarrhoea. For easy consumption by younger children both hips and petals are often made into jellies. Rosehips are useful for all minor infections and bladder problems, for stress and fever in the form of rosehip syrup and, as an oil, for burns and scars. In fact, renewed research and commercial interests have recently found that all wild rosehip oil may be appropriate for medicinal use. In Russia rosehips are also used to aid the flow of bile into the duodenum and for liver and kidney disease and bladder inflammation, and as a vasodilator for heart problems and high blood pressure. Moreover, Russian folkloric healers use the plant to treat symptoms of dysentery, rheumatism and inflammation of the spinal nerve roots. Russian research recently found rose petals to have radioprotective effects, which may be useful to those undergoing radiotherapy.

Rosehips contain up to 1.25 per cent vitamin C as well as many other vitamins and minerals, plus protective antioxidant phenols and flavonoids. The petals, as well as the hips, contain anticarcinogenic anthocyanins. Research has found that rosehips have antibacterial, anti-inflammatory and cytotoxic effects (the latter useful in cancer treatment), and most recently that rosehip extract offers an as yet unexplained alleviation of the pain and flexibility problems of osteoarthritis.

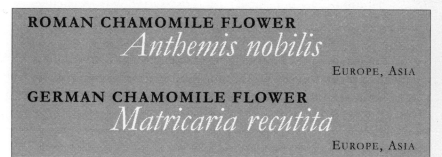

ROMAN CHAMOMILE FLOWER
Anthemis nobilis

EUROPE, ASIA

GERMAN CHAMOMILE FLOWER
Matricaria recutita

EUROPE, ASIA

The name 'chamomile' is derived from the Greek *chamos*, 'ground', and *melos*, 'apple'. The herb has appeared in medical texts since ancient times and was an important drug in Egyptian, Greek and Roman medicines. In Ayurvedic medicine, both Roman and German chamomile are used for respiratory, digestive and nervous disorders. In Russian and Western herbal medicine, German chamomile is used to relieve pain, to calm nerves, to counteract inflammation and as a tonic. Roman chamomile is current in the *British Herbal Pharmacopoeia* for the treatment of dyspepsia, nausea, anorexia, vomiting in pregnancy, dysmenorrhoea and flatulent dyspepsia associated with mental stress.

The flower's essential oil is considered to be an analgesic and to offer many other health benefits. For example, German chamomile's oil is anti-allergenic, anti-inflammatory and antipyretic. In German paediatric medicine, chamomile preparations are the first choice in caring for the sensitive skin of infants and young children, especially for inflammatory skin conditions such as nappy rash and milk crust. The oil is also antispasmodic, bactericidal and fungicidal, and stimulates leucocyte production.

Commercial interest in the herb has led to a lot of scientific research. One study concluded that the flavonoids in chamomile counteract inflammation because they are absorbed deep into the skin. Chamomile ointments have been shown to be as effective as hydrocortisone in the treatment of nerve-related skin rashes, while studies of the use of aromatherapy in childbirth have found that chamomile is effective in alleviating pain. Moreover, the herb's constituent apigenin looks to be promising in inhibiting skin cancers.

Chamomiles are not suitable for those suffering from allergies to the daisy family, and those prescribed metronidazole, anticoagulant or anti-platelet drugs must exercise caution in order to avoid adverse drug interactions. Chamomile oil (*A. nobilis*) is restricted in some countries and the tea may have an effect on the metabolising enzymes in drugs prescribed for liver disorders.

AMERICAN GINSENG
Panax quinquefolius
NEW WORLD

Whether it was the botanist John Bartram or the missionary Father François Lafitu who first found the local people making use of this plant, its rediscovery by Europeans in the first half of the eighteenth century resulted in a Klondike-style rush across the northern states of America. Export to China, where it was used as a yin tonic (mainly for the young) and to treat feebleness, fever and wheezing coughs, was so massive that a century later the plant was heading for extinction in the wild. And this was happening despite the fact that people were already in the habit of saving seeds for replanting. These days American ginseng is cultivated in the USA, China and France. Although proven to be highly antioxidant, this bitter-sweet tonic herb is milder than its Chinese counterpart (see p. 155) and is used mainly to manage stress. Traditionally both herbs have been used to build stamina, enhance cognition and mental acuity, normalise endocrine functions and inhibit the growth of tumours.

Now, research goes on apace on many aspects of this all-American herb. Perhaps the most encouraging to date is a pilot study reported in the *Journal of Psychiatry and Neuroscience* in 2001 on its use for children suffering from attention-deficit hyperactivity disorder (ADHD). Using herbal extract of four parts American ginseng to one part ginkgo (see p. 245) patients were instructed not to change any other medications they were taking during the study. After four weeks' treatment, the proportion of patients showing signs of improvement was 74 per cent as measured on the standard ADHD index and 44 per cent as far as social problems were concerned. Five (14 per cent) out of thirty-six patients reported adverse effects, only two of which were considered to be related to the study medication. It's early days, but it is to be hoped that these preliminary results suggesting that the treatment may alleviate symptoms of ADHD will encourage further research on the use of American ginseng and ginkgo extracts for this purpose.

Medical herbalists warn that American ginseng may not be used in pregnancy, while the list of other contraindications grows as more research is carried out. It may not be used with hypogly-caemic drugs because it intensifies the hypoglycaemic effect; with frusemide because it decreases the diuretic effect; with monoamine oxidase inhibitors (may cause headache, visual hallu-cination, tremor, etc.); with anticoagulants or anti-platelet agents (it decreases the effectiveness of warfarin); or with estogens or corticosteroids (because of drug-combination effects).

DILL

Anethum graveolens

EUROPE

Dill is a biblical herb first recorded in the Ebers papyrus (c. 1500 BC). A pain-killer, dill stems were found on the mummy of the pharaoh Amenophis II. Roman gladiators are said to have rubbed dill oil on their skins before a fight, and the herb was praised in medieval times for reducing sexual impulses. It has been known by its modern name 'dill', which may come from the Norwegian word *dilla* meaning 'to lull', since only the seventeenth century. Today dill's forte is put to best use in gripe water. 'Gripe water', a generic name, has been in worldwise use for generations to relieve some of the symptoms associated with colic, which about 25 per cent of babies suffer from. Traditionally gripe water was made in the kitchen by pouring boiling water over dill seeds.

On the subcontinent of India dill is regarded as a 'cooling' carminative herb, and it is largely employed in cookery. Dill seeds are chewed after meals to aid digestion and sweeten the breath. The herb is known worldwide for promoting the flow of breast milk, and is used to alleviate appetite loss, bronchitis, and liver and gall-bladder problems. In Russia the powdered seeds are used to treat early symptoms of hypertonia (the abnormal tension of arteries or muscles). Its essential oil is useful as a destressant; and American sportsmen 'chill with dill' and use the green brine to toughen the skin.

Recent research has found that both treated and natural dill leaf extract can reduce cholesterol and other lipid levels by 20–50 per cent. The herb's oil, which may not be taken internally, is antimicrobial, and the plant has been shown to have interesting anti-cancer properties.

SAUSAGE TREE
Kigelia africana syn K. pinnata
AFRICA

The Sausage Tree is named after its bitter tasting sausage-like fruits that can be over 2ft. long. It is from these fruits that a dark brown healing extract is derived. Many generations of African healers have made medicines from the roots, bark and fruits of the plant. One application is to use unripe slices of the fruit as a poultice for sores, infested bites and syphilis. In traditional medicine the plant has been mostly applied to problems of the kidney and stomach, but it has many other applications including for worms and wounds. In East Africa, the beverage 'uki' is made from the fruit and the powdered dried bark is used as an antimicrobial dressing for skin infections and as an anti-inflammatory for rheumatism. In the 19th Century British chemists developed a gentle emollient formula from the plant that was successful in helping to improve a variety of long standing dry skin problems. Today, an extract of the plant kigekine is incorporated into skin care and repair products such as exfoliating firming masks and breast enhancing creams. Excellent results have also been obtained using the seed pod cream for eczema especially in children.

International research has indicated positive results with seed pod activity against urinary tract, mouth, lung, intestine, vagina, skin and nail infections. It's emollient extract fights cancerous sun spots and can counter early stages of skin cancer (it contains lapachol, the same anticancer that is found in Pau D'arco). It also contains iridiods, which can show antimicrobial activity in the presence of a hydrolytic (diluted) agent. Stembark aqueous extracts also show inhibitory activity against urinary tract, mouth, lung, intestine, vagina, skin and nail infections.

20

Geriatrics – or, The Survival of the Least Fit

As *Homo sapiens* is, as far as we know, the only product of creative evolution that can learn from history, perhaps in this penultimate chapter I might be allowed to delve once more into those more recent chapters of the saga of herbal medicine.

It was back in the days of Flower Power when Dr Bach's flower formulae were in the ascendant that a rich young businessman tested the bullish herbal health market. Fred Pestalozzi had fallen ill with Ménière's disease (which causes dilation of the labyrinth of the ear, producing bouts of vertigo). He had been prescribed a terminal lifestyle, but hearing of a wonder herbal yeast tonic and with nothing but debilitating time to lose, he tried it – and was cured. Resprouting from a life in the machine-tool business, he set up the company Bio-Strath to make and market a whole range of herbal remedies to the world. A businessman at heart, he did his research and development with scientific precision, and it showed astonishingly good results and few side-effects. Because his products were all tried and tested folk remedies and perhaps because the ghost of Paracelsus still walked the herb-rich alpine pastures of Switzerland, he found no problems in marketing the full range, despite the maze of cantonal rules and regulations through which he had to find his way.

However, as soon as he attempted to market his products abroad – especially in Britain and the USA – difficulties arose. The diehard chemotherapists there, perhaps over-impressed by the ongoing sub-judices of the thalidomide affair and by the nitpickers of herbal rhetoric, joined forces to delay the acceptance of Pestalozzi's products. As with the drugs they were marketing – or peddling, depending from whose side you were viewing the situation — success bred the melancholy of contempt, as it has done throughout the history of herbal medicine. Vested interests — some for money reasons, some craving power and glory, and many out of jealousy fuelled by the fire of divergent opinion — shot their self-styled opponents in the back, and themselves and the whole symbiotic medicine movement in the foot.

The intricacies and inadequacies of the arguments for and against either side make pretty depressing reading, and rarely do we see any standing back and taking stock of the advances on the other side. Bad news has always made headlines, while good news, tainted by the zealots of malpractice, has been relegated to the lower column inches. When in campaigning mode, people often have problems telling the truth, let alone the whole truth and nothing but the truth. (The same goes when they are hell-bent on selling drugs or newspapers.) Anyway, let's try.

Today many humans across a broad range of countries and societies are living longer and without the constant fear of painful remedies being prescribed for their ills, or of a painful death. There are still the ravages of congenital disease, accidents caused by new lifestyles and problems brought on by new diseases. Yet there is no getting away from the fact that, despite all those food additives and the ever-spreading rash of articles about illness for readers to digest, more and more people survive to reproduce. Also, more live on, fraught with the syndromes of old age — arthritis, rheumatism, Alzheimer's disease, and of course cancer in all its manifestations.

Unfortunately, or perhaps fortunately, none of the elixirs of long life that have been 'discovered' to date keeps the ageing process permanently at bay — whether it's the muscles, the skin, the joints, the bones or the brain, or all of them, that are under attack. It's hardly surprising, then, that today more and more of our hospital beds are occupied by victims of geriatric syndromes, of replacement or cosmetic surgery, or of iatrogenics — that is, the diseases or symptoms induced by the treatment prescribed for underlying disorders. The survival of the least fit is now a growth industry on a First World scale, and the unfit are getting younger all the time.

Recycling of the gene stock at regular intervals has served the human species well over its short existence. New bodies for old has been the way of natural selection, honing the fit towards fitness for survival and dragging the unfit, along with all the pathogens, towards extinction. The problem now is that with a world population of over six billion that has the potential to recycle itself at an ever-increasing rate – thanks to science, the pharmaceutical industry, medicine and, yes, the age-old and now reworked materia medica – our success now threatens to kill the golden goose. The biosphere is dying thanks to the devices, desires and aspirations of this exploding population, destroying as it goes the very hope we have for survival, let alone the healthful lifestyle we all crave. Good food in moderation and in the right combination, not too much work, play of the right sort and a spacious, airy place to live, as advocated in the Talmud written twenty-three centuries ago, still seems the way ahead.

The most terrible indictment of today's hi-tech multimedia society is that in every twenty-four hours one hundred thousand people, give or take a few, die of conditions relating to malnutrition and environmental pollution – in simple terms, die of starvation and dirty water. It was put most eloquently by Robert McNamara, one-time president of the World Bank, when he reminded the world that 25 per cent of the world's population live in 'a condition of life so characterised by malnutrition, illiteracy, disease, high infant mortality and low life expectancy as to be beneath any reasonable definition of human decency'. But the amazing reality is that, thanks to the resilience of the human genome, the advances of sanitation and agricultural, medical and pharmaceutical science as well as the great band of traditional herbalists working away in the undergrowth from which they glean their wonder drugs, 250,000 arrive to swell the global breakfast table of each new day. A quarter of a million new mouths to feed, new bodies to be clothed, housed, and medically serviced, the vast majority still thanks to herbal-based medicine.

Little wonder, then, that despite the smouldering antagonism of much of the medical profession, the World Health Organisation in 1974 announced that 'in order to reach the goal of adequate health care for everyone by the year 2000' part of their policy would be to encourage all Third World countries to develop their own traditional systems of medicine. Four years later they recommended that 'each country . . . begin systematic study of their medicinal plants, the accent being on whole-plant drugs'.

Twenty-nine long years have passed since then – twenty-nine years during which each minute has seen the premature death of at least seventy people and — wait for it — the destruction of some 60 hectares of natural vegetation. How many potential Einsteins or Te Kanawas, and how many potentially useful plant species have we lost? To date, less than 1 per cent of plant species have been investigated by modern science, and as the forests recede so too does the knowledge of indigenous tribal people. Take note of the facts revealed by Brian M. Boom of the New York Botanical Garden. In a study of the Chacobo people of Bolivia he ascertained that they were finding uses for 75 species or 619 individual trees, in a sample hectare containing 649 trees of 94 species; that's to say, they were finding uses for 82 per cent of the total species available on their patch, and for 95 per cent of the individual trees. The species were grouped into five classes according to use: food, fuel, crafts and construction, medicinal and commercial. Some species, especially the palms, fell into more than one category.

Ladies and gentlemen, this is our last chance. The living world of which we know we are a part is dying from an iatrogenic disease caused by a pathogen called *Homo sapiens*, which is destroying the life-support system of the earth and the best-stocked pharmacy there has ever been. If the medical profession in all its twenty-first-century guises can't see that their way ahead is via a new, eclectic approach, with the best of the old working in symbiosis with the best of the new to solve the real problems of what could be, if we don't do something about it, then the future of humankind hasn't a chance.

We must use the greenprint of medicare handed down to the West over more than sixty thousand years to grasp a very reachable and respectable goal: every child a wanted child, a healthy child, growing up into an individual who can aspire to the dignity inherent in being a member of a truly civilised world, and an average active life of perhaps a little more than three score years and ten. So leading on to an active old age, not *sans* eyes, *sans* teeth, *sans* everything, but *sans* the pain and the anguish of iatrogenic and geriatric syndromes.

PADMA 28
Complex of many herbs
ASIA

Tibetan medicine, which is over 2,500 years old, is based on maintaining the 'harmony of nature's organisms' – not a bad definition of the importance of biodiversity. Many remedies, such as the potent antioxidant herbal complex 'Padma 28', are based on a blend of plants aimed at restoring balance to the body. Padma 28 is used for problems of the arms and legs, including tension and loss of feeling. It can be traced back two thousand years, but was only rediscovered, researched and championed by a Swiss pharmaceutical entrepreneur, Karl Lutz, in the 1960s. Nineteen of its twenty-two ingredients are herbal, and it is claimed that it is the combination rather than any one ingredient in particular that yields the desired balancing effect.

Research has found that Padma 28 is useful in intermittent claudication (characterised by a cramp-like pain in the legs), the symptoms of which range from pins and needles to total immobility, and that it can help those affected to walk less painfully. Other studies have pointed to the mixture's high concentrations and balance of antioxidants as a modulator of the immune system. With 2.6 million people in the UK alone suffering from intermittent claudication, the treatment of which can involve delicate and expensive surgery, it looks as if interest will remain high in Padma 28.

JAPANESE KNOTWEED
Polygonum multiflorum
EUROPE, ASIA

Fo ti, a cousin of the ultra-invasive Japanese knotweed, has been used in China for thousands of years, where it is called the 'elixir of long life'. Originally noted in medical literature in 713 AD, *he shou wu*, meaning 'black-haired mister', is widely used in China for the traditional purpose of restoring black hair and other evidences of youth. With a tonic effect on the kidneys and liver, this herb is said to keep one vigorous and to extend the human lifespan. According to traditional Chinese medicine, it builds up the blood and sperm and strengthens various other parts of the body, and has been used effectively for insomnia, dizziness and coronary disease amongst other disorders. The whole root has been shown to reduce cholesterol levels and to lower hypertension.

Fo ti is not usually recommended today for people with phlegm or diarrhoea, or those with kidney or liver problems, although in China it is thought to tone up the kidneys and liver. Side-effects are infrequent, mainly limited to mild diarrhoea and rare allergic reaction. Some traditional sources advise that it should not be taken with onions, chives or garlic. Unwanted effects on the liver induced by this herb may well be due to pre-existing physiological deficits in the consumer or to contamination.

ELDERBERRY
Sambucus nigra
EUROPE, ASIA

Known in ancient Greece as 'the tree of musical pipes', the elder has a very long history in folkloric medicine. In Britain the berries are used as an analgesic brew to be taken at the first sign of headache, and they make good cordials and 'tonic' wines. Elderberry syrup has been used down the ages for coughs and colds and upper respiratory tract infections. In Russian folk medicine an infusion of spring leaves and autumn berries is mixed with honey and used to cure chronic constipation, and an extract made of the berries and young shoots is used as a diuretic to treat kidney problems accompanied by oedema. As in the British Isles, the flowers and berries are used to make cake fillings, jam, jellies and sweets that are mildly laxative and useful for people with irritated or inflamed intestines.

In recent years, in an attempt to find an influenza cure, research has started to focus on the antiviral properties of the fruit of black elder. Influenza is an acute illness which causes seventy thousand deaths every year in the USA alone. Laboratory tests in Israel have shown that an anthocyanin-rich elderberry extract called Sambucol protects cells against many different flu viruses. A syrup and a lozenge containing the key active components of Sambucol have cured 90 per cent of the patients in a test group. Recent research has proved that it stimulates and protects the immune system when given to cancer or AIDS patients undergoing chemotherapy or other treatments. These are still early days, but this simple old-fashioned remedy looks set to become a herbal leader in the postmodern world.

ECHINACEA CONEFLOWER
Echinacea spp.

NEW WORLD

Out of nine species of coneflower, three are used medicinally, *E. angustifolia*, *E. purpurea* and *E. pallida*, and were also used by Native Americans, mainly to treat wounds. 'Echinacea' is a term that broadly refers to the extracts derived from both the aerial parts and the roots of these plants. In America, Eclectic physicians used echinacea in the late 1800s and early 1900s, about which time it became popular in Germany. Since those early days, the herb has been adopted into the Ayurvedic system of medicine and is generally used worldwide as an immune-system stimulant; it is also anti-inflammatory, antibiotic, detoxifying, sudorific (sweat-inducing) and anti-allergenic; and it heals wounds.

Echinacea is a unique infection-fighter, very popular as a herbal medicine for colds, flu, viruses and infections of all kinds. In the United States from 1995 to 1998, preparations from various parts of the plant constituted the top-selling herbal medicine in healthfood stores. Early research into these three 'globe flowers' is extremely positive, and the antibacterial and antiviral effects are well documented both in vitro and clinically. In its role as proven immunostimulant echinacea strengthens the body against infections, whether viral or bacterial. Note its unique distinction of being able to attack viruses directly — an asset that permits echinacea to outshine many comparable pharmaceuticals.

Often two, or all three, species of medicinal echinacea have been mixed together, and there has been much debate about the plant's effects and possible side-effects. All three are proven antioxidants, and research has also shown *E. pallida* to have good anti-inflammatory and wound-healing properties. However, one thing is clear: a great deal more research is required to unlock the full power of these amazing herbs.

ROOIBOS TEA
Aspalathus linearis
AFRICA

Rooibos, or rooibosch, is a spiny shrub found only in southern Africa. The Khoikhoi tribe are said to have been the first to use the plant's mahogany-red 'tea leaves' to brew aromatic herbal tea. In the early 1900s rooibos was marketed in South Africa as 'Mountain Tea' and its trade was regulated in the 1950s. Long valued in the region, the health properties of the tea are now becoming recognised internationally and its popularity is increasing rapidly.

The caffeine-free tea has been used to alleviate stomach and digestive problems such as nausea, vomiting, heartburn, stomach ulcers and constipation. Containing no oxalic acid, it may also be drunk freely by those suffering from kidney-stones. The herb's antispasmodic properties relieve stomach cramp and colic in infants, and it has been beneficial in the management of allergies like hay fever, asthma and eczema. At the London Olympia 2001 International Natural Products Exhibition, rooibos had even found its way into cosmetic toiletries. It has a soothing effect on the skin, relieving irritations. It is also useful for those on a restricted diet and is said to aid sleep.

The tea contains flavonoids, polysaccharides, polyphenols and an extremely high level of antioxidants. If it is brewed for longer than ten minutes, its antioxidant effects intensify. It also contains the minerals iron, zinc, potassium, magnesium, calcium, copper, manganese, sodium and fluoride.

Research has found rooibos to be beneficial in the treatment of many disorders that particularly affect the elderly, such as high blood pressure, diabetes mellitus, atherosclerosis, allergic and skin conditions, liver disease and cataracts. Recent studies have also shown that it may have a role to play in anti-cancer and anti-HIV treatment.

NONI, INDIAN MULBERRY
Morinda citrifolia

ASIA

Noni, or Indian mulberry, is a small evergreen tree that grows in open coastal regions and in fairly low-altitude forested areas. It is often found along lava flows, which is why there is an abundance of the plant in Hawaii, said to have been brought to the islands by early Polynesians who migrated there around the time of Christ. Contact with Western diseases brought by Captain Cook and his crew in 1778 decimated the natives of Hawaii, and much of the oral tradition of their healers and herbalists was lost. Fortune has it that noni, about which many traditional healing myths revolved, was one of the 317 medicinal plants that were documented at the time, and we know that its roots, stems, bark, leaves, flowers and fruit were all used.

The leaves and fruits of *M. citrifolia*, also called *ba ji*, are used in India to reduce inflammation, dysentery and haemorrhage, amongst other problems. In China another species, *M. officinalis* (*ba ji tain*), first recorded during the Han dynasty (206 BC – 220 AD), is made into a warming tonic to treat premature ejaculation in men and infertility in both men and women, plus other hormonally linked conditions. It is also used for urinary infirmity, especially incontinence, which is often experienced by the elderly.

In the past decade, people in the West have been using noni for diabetes, high blood pressure, cancer and other illnesses. The herb contains a natural alkaloid that is converted to xeronine in the digestive tract. Incredibly, xeronine is active down to one-trillionth of a gram. Noni also contains many vitamins and minerals. However, it may not be taken by those suffering from hyperkalaemia, a condition characterised by an abnormally high concentration of potassium in the blood, because of its own high potassium content (which can be very useful where renal function is normal). Studies have shown that the herb has sedative and antibacterial properties. It has also been shown to suppress tumour growth indirectly by stimulating the immune system; when the active substance in this process, identified in 1999 as 'noni-ppt', was combined with suboptimal doses of the standard chemotherapeutic agents, it enhanced the curative effects and extended the survival time.

KOMBUCHA TEA
Yeasts, bacteria, tea and sugar
CHINA

The first recorded use of kombucha tea was in China during the Tsin dynasty, when it was referred to as 'the remedy for immortality'. Subsequently it was used throughout China, Japan and Korea, and was later introduced into Russia and India. It resurfaced in Japan between the wars after many healthy hundred-plus-year-olds in the Kargasok region were found to be drinkers of the fermentation. Now it is widely used in Japan.

'Kombucha' is the Germanic rendition of the Japanese name for a membrane consisting of a symbiotic colony of yeast and bacteria, living in a solution of tea and sugar in which it constantly multiplies. It is said that if properly treated it will last a lifetime, and the 'tea fungus', or culture, is often given as a token of friendship. Many positive effects have been experienced by tea-drinkers. Kombucha may, for example, act as a gentle laxative and alleviate problems such as arthritis, stomach cramps and insomnia. It is also claimed to revitalise the body and increase energy.

Russian studies have linked the drinking of the tea with a low incidence of cancer, and recent research in India has shown it to

have potent antimicrobial, antioxidant and immunogenic properties. It is thought that kombucha does not target a specific organ,
but heightens the body's defences against environmental stress.
The yeast feeds on the sugar and produces a wide range of active
substances such as glucuronic acid, which is also found in the
liver, where it binds toxins ready to be expelled.

It could be said that kombucha has mainly suffered a bad press
and a negative attitude on the part of scientific researchers.
However, in 2001 it was found to have no significant toxicity, to
significantly decrease paracetamol poisoning of the liver, and to
have liver-protective and anti-stress properties. Whether the suspected or the proven cases of adverse effects are due to various
forms of contamination of the culture tea rather than from the
tea itself is a subject of debate. Much more positive research into
the tea's remedial potential is desirable.

ARCTIC ROOT
Rhodiola rosea
EURASIA

Arctic root is found naturally in northern regions of Europe and
for thousands of years has been eaten and used in traditional
medicine to give strength and stamina, to treat long-term illness
and debility and as a favoured ingredient in many folk love
potions. The Russian government has for years given Arctic root
to its key figures such as athletes, astronauts and politicians to
help improve mental, physical and psychological performance. Its
powers were revealed when the Soviet Union opened its Iron
Curtain to the West. It is one of the most astounding and versatile herbs ever to be studied, modern research highlighting its use
as an adaptogenic anti-stress agent working by increasing the
body's natural resistance to various stresses. It can also increase
the body's capacity for exercise. In short, it is a general tonic for
well-being, and has become very much a twenty-first-century
herb.

Clinical research suggests that compounds found within

Rhodiola increase the amount of serotonin reaching the brain. (Insufficient serotonin can cause depression.) Use of the herb also leads to an increase in the amount of basic beta-endorphin in the blood plasma, which inhibits the hormonal changes indicative of stress. By curbing stress, Arctic root can also help prevent cardiac damage. Some of its ability to affect physical and mental performance is explained by the fact that it increases the amounts of adenosine triphosphate and creatine phosphate in muscle tissue and of fatty acids in the blood. Recently, researchers have discovered that the plant has slimming properties, and it is also being investigated for men suffering from weak erection and premature ejaculation.

AMRIT KALASH
Ayurvedic herbal formula

Amrit kalash was developed thousands of years ago by the Ayurvedic sages as a formula for total health. The herbal remedy was used as an antidote to tiredness and included in a routine combining hatha yoga exercises, nutritious meals and herbal teas. Contemporary scientific studies indicate a wide range of benefits offered by *Amrit kalash*. These include the retardation of premature ageing, an increase in alertness, a sharpening of focus, a reduction in fatigue and stress and heightened energy.

Extensive research has shown that *amrit kalash* is a complete, 'full-spectrum', antioxidant that can eliminate all of the hundreds of types of free radicals that are thought to be the underlying cause of over 70 per cent of all disease. It has been shown to have a thousand times more antioxidant power than vitamins C or E, the vitamins that many of us take as supplements in a bid to neutralise free radicals in order to stay healthy.

The Ayurvedic food supplement MAK (*maharishi amrit kalash*) has been shown to have the potential to compensate for any decline in antioxidant enzymes in the central nervous system, thereby reducing the risk of lipid peroxidation. This means that it could play a role in rejuvenating the ageing central nervous system's antioxidant defence system. Various forms of MAK may be useful in the prevention and treatment of atherosclerosis. It has also been shown to modulate the immune system, to inhibit the growth of melanomas (skin cancers), and to reverse some of the adverse cognitive effects of ageing.

STOP PRESS

Recent work at Harvard Medical School indicates that a diet rich in vitamin E foods could help fight off Parkinson's disease, while a study by the National Institute of Ageing in Chicago suggests that such a diet may reduce the risk of developing Alzeimer's disease by 67 per cent. The best sources are olive oil, hazelnuts, broccoli and almonds.

Postscripts
for Sustainable People

GENETIC ENGINEERING, STEM CELLS AND CLONING

When you were a fertilised egg, you were a single totipotent stem cell. Totipotency means that, with the basic set of information you received from Mum and Dad, that single cell could divide again and again, eventually producing 100 trillion cells of the 230 different types that go to make you.

Your one cell divided into two, then two into four, all of which were stem cells and hence totipotent, still capable of producing another complete you. (That's how identical twins and quads happen.) From that point on, more and more of the cells lost their Jack-and-Jill-of-all-trades totipotency. The outer layer of the expanding ball of cells went to make up your mum's placenta and other parts of your life support system, while the dividing mass inside became less and less totipotent. Each cell continued to divide, taking on an ever more specialised role: the production of your blood, brains, kidneys, and all your other particular bits. How all this is accomplished we have little idea, but if it didn't happen we would end up as a giant bag of potentially cancerous cells. The exciting thing is that in the normal course of events it all works out, and a unique bonny bouncing baby is born.

Recent research has shown that even in the ageing adult, stem cells have the ability, given the right conditions, to divide and still to produce a whole range of different cells. This enables the creation of a brand-new bit of liver, lung, kidney or muscle unique to you, and so bringing with it none of the problems of rejection by your body as happens with organs transplanted from other donors. Organ transplants are without doubt one of the greatest success stories of twentieth-century medical science. It must be borne in mind, though, that the many patients who receive organs from donors other than their identical siblings have to remain for the rest of their lives on a complex of medicaments that reduce the possibility of rejection. But it's a small price to pay for all those extra active years.

The potential exists, however, with the help of ethical science and an ethical health system, for a 'grow your own new bits and pieces ready for use in emergency' service to be researched and put into operation. No need to use stem cells from aborted embryos, which come with the added complication of ethics, let alone rejection by the patient as a foreign body; or to have to contemplate the ultimate horror, that the foreign embryonic or other organ would turn into a cancerous growth. (This has in fact already happened in the case of some foreign stem cell experiments with volunteers suffering from Parkinson's disease. In contrast, experiments using people's own stem cells have given promising results.)

And to cap it all, apparently straight out of sci-fi emerges the possibility of having your body frozen – cryogenically stored and ready for rejuvenation when the elixir of life – or anyway a method far beyond the ultimate body lift – has been discovered.

So why, one must ask, isn't it all-systems-go to set such a replacement-parts system in motion? Well, the problem is finding who'll pay for the very expensive research. Pharmaceutical companies have investors who want more than their pound of annual dividend back before they die. So the end product must be patentable. Already unethical patents have been applied for and some, unfortunately, obtained on particular genetic traits of tribal people in different parts of the world. The difficulty is that patenting one person's stem cells for potential use on him or herself would be rightly regarded as a dead-end investment. Also, without the need for all those drugs till death parts you from your borrowed bits and pieces, share prices might tumble. I apologise if I am treading on anyone's toes, but somewhere in all this mess there must be an answer, and I hope ethics may raise its head soon and solve the problem.

AID AND AIDS

All the evidence gathered to date indicates that HIV, the human immunodeficiency virus, evolved by chance somewhere in Africa in the early 1940s. Sixty years on the *Herald Tribune*, three days after Christmas 2001, carried a front-page headline in a black box proclaiming 'Africans Plead in Vain for AIDS Treatment'. The article outlined how a potential solution, at least, to the suffering caused by the retroviral disease started with a meeting in Geneva in 1991 concerning global access to AIDS drugs, and how despite promises from leading international companies, a decade later nothing of note had happened. Now twenty-five million people in Africa are doomed to die a terrible death because neither the corporate world nor the aid agencies have been willing or able to rock the global economy to make aid for AIDS available on a massive enough scale.

I could be wrong in my interpretation of the article, but between the lines at least twice it seemed to be saying that, like most things in the world, it comes down to money. The only real hope offered came from one Dr Pronyk in an interview outside the Elite Funeral Parlor, the only thriving business in view from his office at the hospital where he has been researching the problem: 'We've got to look further upstream, to stop all the new people from falling in. Otherwise the people drowning now are going to be endlessly replaced.' Then came the warning that 'at current levels of intervention, the number of Africans dead of AIDS in ten years will hit 60 million' – 1 per cent of the then total world population.

You can buy a lot of condoms for $10,000, the going rate for the new retroviral drugs to keep one AIDS patient alive for one year. In biological terms it doesn't really matter because despite rampant malnutrition, environmental pollution and AIDS, as noted earlier there are 250,000 extra mouths to be fed every day, mainly from the crumbs that fall from the fast-food tables of the world. So the species is in no immediate danger, and neither are the dividends of the shareholders of the processed-food and pharmaceutical companies. But in humanitarian terms? Well, turning back to the article in the *Herald Tribune*:

Mr Merson said in a recent interview that an early visit to Uganda seared itself into his memory. He touched down in Kampala on

2 September 1990, for talks with the government. But Noerine Kaleeba, a local pioneer in AIDS community care, talked him into an impromptu call on her clinic. Mr Merson was stunned at the sight of stick-figure patients dying on floors, unable to swallow because of fungal infections, unmedicated for their pain and 'begging, begging for help'.

That was over a decade ago, and the world is still arguing what to do about it.

If only humanity could agree to forget its other differences and reshape its ever more sophisticated and expensive weapons of war into the ploughshares of cheap retroviral medicines or, better still, vaccines, backed up, of course, by modern reproductive and nutritional healthcare. The only question left to answer would be how to maintain the mortgages and lifestyles of the investors and employees of the arms industry. And one last thing: if the prognostications on global warming are right, the potential rise in sea level is not going to help matters at coastal cities, many of them powerhouses of global trade; along with much of the world's most productive agricultural land, they cannot fail to be threatened with inundation.

DRUMSTICK TREE
Moringa oleifera

AFRICA, ASIA

Moringa is perhaps today best known for its powdered seeds, used to purify water in West Africa. However, in this modern world, wherever there are dirty water and malnutrition the diseases that go with them usually stalk the land. The fast-growing moringa, the drumstick or horseradish tree, used to be grown to produce ben oil (a lubricant for watches and for salads), and in tropical climes it has long been regarded as a famine food. It is now being put through its paces in the Sahel region of Africa, between the advancing Sahara and what's left of the savannah forests, which are in massive retreat. This is a region of the world in which famine has become endemic, since village life has for many reasons been blighted by absolute poverty.

All parts of the drumstick tree are edible: leaf, leaf powder, flowers, pods, seeds, roots and bark, all of which are good sources of protein, vitamins, minerals and metals. In some countries such as Niger it is already grown as a cash crop. Moringa leaves can be cooked like spinach, used to make a sauce and served over rice or couscous, or easily dried into a powder and stored for long periods. Young pods can be cooked like green beans. Older pods, seeds, flowers, roots and bark are also considered tasty.

Research has proved that charcoal from this tree when dissolved in water and drunk removes the liver toxin, microcystin-LR. This discovery has spurred research into other aspects of this miracle tree, not least in so far as what it can do for the immune system and against HIV/AIDS. The nutritional powerhouse that is the moringa leaf has been found to have four times the vitamin A content of carrots, which helps to fortify the immune system, building resistance to diseases such as malaria as well as HIV/AIDS. It also contains vitamin E, amino acids and fatty acids, and minerals including calcium, iron, copper and zinc (in large amounts).

Moringa seed oil (called mbololo seed oil in Kenya) has been found to contain 'high levels of unsaturated fatty acids, especially oleic' (up to 75.39 per cent). The oil was also found to be rich in plant sterols and tocopherols. Apart from containing antioxidants, the oil also showed resistance to rancidity – that is, good storage potential.

Although the main focus of interest in moringa has been its great nutritional value, research tells us that it has infinitely more to offer. The leaves also contain alkaloids that promote liver and kidney function and that, at low dosage, do not produce adverse effects; and in research in Pakistan moringa pods have shown potential for use in hypertension. Philippino plant researchers have found that the leaves contain a compound, tested in vitro and in vivo in mice, that may prevent cancers from forming. And the Japanese have shown this compound be effective against

Epstein-Barr virus. The leaf extract may be used to regulate hyperthyroidism, and shows promise as a cholesterol-reducer. Not least, used in mice before whole-body exposure to radiation, it suggests that survival might be possible for up to thirty days – which holds important implications for us humans in our nuclear world.

The planting of a few billion of these trees not only holds out the promise of slowing the advance of the Sahara, it would put food medicine and pure water into the stomachs of the millions awaiting the next hand-out of aid (or AIDS), while sequestering the carbon that could give the global greenhouse the breathing space that the Kyoto countries are gasping for.

This represents, of course, only a small part of the research being carried out on this truly amazing tree, spearheaded not by a pharmaceutical giant but by the Christian World Service. CWS has already published a book, *The Miracle Tree*, and plans to convene an international conference on the subject. The only thing holding up the progress of this crucially important work is lack of funds.

Two plants have emerged out of the heritage of Africa that may have the potential to cure many ills: moringa, just described, is putting not only pure water and nutritious food, but also hope, into some of the poorest people of the world, while the long-kept secret of the Hoodia cactus, cultivated by the Bushmen of the Kalahari, may soon be solving the plumptious problems of some of the world's richest people. Surely it would not be drawing too heavily on the milk (soya it may be) of human kindness for those that can, to begin to share the rights of intellectual profit. Surely, in these days of instant communication nations should – and rapidly – learn to speak more than peace unto nation.

Glossary

Adaptogen: Aiding adaptation of the body, improving resistance, particularly to stress.

ADHD: Attention-Deficit Hyperactivity Disorder (in children) denoting short attention span, unruly behaviour etc. Some potential causes are thought to occur via dietary food additives termed 'E's, colourants and azo dyes e.g. E102 Tartrazine.

Adrenal glands: Two triangular glands, covering the superior surface of each kidney, secreting several steroid hormones.

Alginate: A substance obtained from seaweeds often used as thickening in foods.

Alkaloid: One of a diverse group of nitrogen-containing organic substances naturally produced by plants and having potent effect on body function.

Allopathy: The orthodox system of medicine, in which the use of drugs is directed to produce effects in the body to alleviate the symptoms of a disease.

Alpha-carotene: One of four forms of carotenoids (alpha-, beta-, gamma- and delta-) that are yellow or orange coloured pigments found in plants, e.g. beta-carotene.

Alternative: Relating to Complementary Medicine, it describes various systems of healing that are not regarded as part of orthodox treatment by the medical profession. Some disciplines are now accepted, e.g. osteopathy.

Amine: (Aminoalkanes) Organic derivatives of ammonia that are part of the amino group and are an essential component of the amino acids.

Amino acid: (Aminoalkanoic acids) Fundamental constituents that are the basic structure units of all proteins. Essential amino acids must be obtained from protein in the diet.

Anabolic: Promoting tissue growth by increasing the metabolic processes involved in protein synthesis. Anabolic agents are usually synthetic male sex hormones – used to assist weight gain and to strengthen the bones in osteoporosis. Some may cause virilisation (masculinity) in women and liver damage.

Anaphylaxis: An abnormal reaction to a particular antigen, in which histamine is released from tissues and causes either local or widespread symptoms, e.g. an allergic attack is a localized anaphylaxis; anaphylactic shock is an extreme generalised allergic reaction.

Anodyne: Soothes and eases pain.

Anthocyanin: A potent antioxidant protector, red/blue-purple pigments found in fruits, e.g. raspberries, blueberries and plums, and in other foods, e.g. nasunin in aubergine.

Antigen: Any substance the body regards as alien or potentially dangerous, against which it produces an antibody.

Antioxidant: Prevents or hinders the deterioration of cells by oxidation.

Antipyretic: Alleviates fever.

Antussive: Relieves cough.

Arachidic acid: An essential fatty acid, e.g. found in apricot kernel and borage oils.

Arrhythmia: Any deviation from the normal rhythm (sinus rhythm) of the heart.

Astringent: Causing contraction of the tissues; binding, which effect reduces bleeding and discharges.

Arteriosclerosis: Loss of elasticity in the artery walls due to thickening and calcification.

Atherosclerosis: A disease of the arteries in which fatty plaques develop on their inner walls, causing eventual obstruction of blood flow.

'B':

Beta-carotene: The yellow/orange plant pigment that is converted in the body to vitamin A, e.g. found in apricots and oranges.

Betaine: A chemical atom, an ion, carrying both a positive and a negative charge, occurring naturally in plants and mammals, e.g. present in solid and liquid amino acids such as glycin.

Bioavailability: Available to living organisms such as the human body.

Bioflavonoid: Usually refers to a plant flavonoid freely available to the human body.

Biogeochemical: An earth chemical available to living organisms that follows the principles governing the geological distribution of individual elements.

Biomarker: A marker used to fix or help to trace and aid analysis of the progress of chemical processes in living organisms.

Bioresorbable: The process of resorption, i.e. loss of substance through physiological or pathological means in living organisms; e.g. uric acid when not expelled from the body in urine may be reabsorbed back into the body to form uric crystals in joints, causing inflammations and pain such as gout.

'C':

Calciferol: Vitamin D, involved in calcium and phosphorous metabolism.

Carcinogen: Any substance or radiation, natural or synthetic, that causes
cancer.

Cardiostimulant: Stimulates the heart.

Carminative: Warming, relieves flatulence.

Carotene: A yellow or orange plant pigment – one of the carotenoids.

Carotenoid: Any one of a group of about 100 naturally occurring yellow to red pigments found mostly in plants, including carotenes.

Casein: A milk protein, e.g. it is the principal protein of cheese, useful as a supplement in the treatment of malnutrition.

Chemopreventive: Chemical or chemistry preventing disease.

Chemotherapeutic: Treatment or healing of disease by the use of chemical substances.

CLA (Conjugated Linoleic Acid): A fatty acid shown potentially to be a key factor in weight management, e.g. found in sunflower.

Collagen: A protein that is the principal constituent of white fibrous connective tissue with high tensile strength, found in skin, cartilage, tendons, ligaments and bone.

Corpuscles: Usually refers to blood corpuscles.

Corpus luteum: Glandular tissue formed at the site of a ruptured follicle after ovulation that secretes the hormone progesterone, preparing the womb for implantation.

Corticosteroid: Any steroid hormone synthesised by the adrenal cortex, e.g. hydrocortisone.

Coumarin: A plant constituent that is used in perfumes and flavour-
ings, and in remedies as a drug to prevent coagulation (blood clotting).

Cyanogenic: Pertaining to cyanide production, e.g. occurring in seeds
of bitter almonds.

Cytoplasm: The living contents of all cells excluding the nucleus and
other major structures.

Cytotoxic: Able to kill cells, e.g. cytotoxic T-lymphocytes.

'D':

Demulcent: Substances that soothe and protect mucous membranes
and relieve irritation.

Dermis: The true skin – a thick layer of living tissue beneath the epidermis, consisting of mainly loose connective tissue, containing
blood capillaries, lymph vessels, sensory nerve endings, sweat
glands and their ducts, hair follicles, sebaceous glands and smooth
muscle fibres.

Digitalis: A very poisonous extract from the dried leaves of foxgloves
(Digitalis species) used to treat heart failure.

DNA (Deoxyribonucleic acid): The genetic material of nearly all living
organisms that controls heredity and is located in the cell nucleus.

DVT (Deep Vein Thrombosis): a condition currently associated with
attacks sustained due to inactivity when airborne for long periods.

'E':

The Eclectic tradition: In the late 18th and early 19th centuries in
America and Britain various pioneers practiced 'eclectic' medicine,
selecting ideas or beliefs from a variety of sources. These incorporated different disciplines, e.g. botanical medicine and phrenology,
to treat the many diseases prevalent in urban societies.

Elastin: Protein forming the major constituent of elastic tissue fibres.

Emollient: Soothes and softens skin.

Endocrine gland system: Ductless glands that manufacture one or
more hormones and secrete them directly into the bloodstream,
including the pituitary, thyroid, parathyroid, adrenal glands, the
ovary and testis, the placenta, and part of the pancreas.

Endorphin: One of a group of chemical compounds that occur naturally in the brain and have pain-relieving properties similar to those

of the opiates.

Endosperm: Plant tissue formed within the embryo-sac, serving in the nutrition of the embryo and often increasing to form a storage tissue in the mature seed.

Endotherm: A chemical reaction associated with the absorption of heat. Also a warm blooded animal.

Enteric: Relating to or affecting the intestine.

Enzyme: A protein that in small amounts speeds up the rate of biological reaction without itself being used up in the reaction. It acts as a catalyst.

Ester: A chemical compound formed by the interaction of an acid and an alcohol. e.g. many esters have a fruity smell and are used in artificial fruit essences or as solvents.

'F':

FDA: The American Food and Drugs Administration. Equivalent to the British MCA (Medicines Control Agency).

Febrifuge: Reduces fever.

Fixed (of oil): Plant oils used as carrier oils in aromatherapy and massage are termed 'fixed' oils because they do not evaporate, are not soluble in alcohol, and essential oils easily dissolve in them, e.g. sweet almond and coconut oils.

Folate: Another name for folic acid, also called folacin. It is a unit of nutritive value classed as a vitamin found in milk and milk products with traces in meat and meat products and in fats and oils. Also found in fruits and vegetables, they are highly available in nuts, e.g. almonds and cashews.

Folic acid (Pteroglutamic acid): Another name for water-soluble vitamin B_9, part of the B complex of vitamins.

Food Medicine: Food is not only a source of nutrition; it provides all the vitamins and minerals the body requires to function. Foods also contain important active compounds and properties that may be classed as 'medicine', e.g. nutritious blueberries assist the construction of collagen.

Fractionated oil: Fractionatal distillation (of oils) is a process used for the separation of various components of liquid mixtures and, e.g. in the case of commercially available coconut oil, to remove harmful compounds.

Free radicals: Groups of atoms containing unpaired electrons that are capable of free existence usually only for very short periods, but are considered to cause damage to living cells through oxidation. The free radical reaction involves the loss of electrons from paired atoms resulting in their reduction or loss.

'G':

GLA (Gamma-linolenic acid): A fatty acid occurring naturally in breast milk, borage and evening primrose oils which can also be produced in the body from linoleic acid.

Glucosamine (Glucosamine sulphate): The amino sugar of glucose that is a nutrient found in very small amounts in food, also made by cartilage cells of the body. It mainly activates the production of glycoaminoglycans (GSGs) required to construct cartilage.

Glucose (Dextrose): A simple sugar found in the blood or in e.g. grapes, an important source of energy to the body and sole source of energy for the brain.

Glutathione: A peptide containing the amino acids glutamic acid, cysteine, and glycine, functioning as a co-enzyme in several oxidation-reduction reactions.

Gluten: A mixture of two proteins, gliadin and glutenin, it is present in wheat and rye and is important for its baking properties. Sensitivity to gluten leads to celiac disease.

Glycosides: A group of compounds, including glucosides, derived from other monosaccharides, e.g. glucose.

'H':

HDL (High-Density Lipoprotein): A type of blood fat that helps to prevent cholesterol deposits from settling in the arteries.

Hepatic: Relating to the liver.

Hepatocyte: The principal cell type in the liver with metabolic functions, including synthesis, storage, detoxification and bile production.

Heroic medicine: A system of urban oriented medicine that relied on the

administration of poisons, common around the period of the Industrial Revolution when practice of rural medicine began to decline.

Homoeopathy: A system of medicine based on the theory that 'like cures like', founded by Samuel Hahnemann (1755-1843).

Hyperlipidaemia: The presence in the blood of an abnormally high concentration of fats.

Hypoglycaemia: A reduction of sugar (glucose) in the blood, causing muscular weakness, inco-ordination, mental confusion and sweating.

Hypotension: Abnormally low blood pressure.

Hypothalamus: A part of the brain controlling body temperature, thirst, hunger, eating, water balance and sexual function etc.

'I':

Iatrogenic: Describing a condition that has resulted from treatment as either an unforeseen or inevitable side-effect.

Immunostimulant: A substance or something that stimulates the immune system.

Insulin: A protein hormone produced in the pancreas by the beta cells of the islets of Langerhans, important for regulating the amount of sugar (glucose) in the blood.

'in vitro': Describing biological phenomena that are made to occur outside the living body – traditionally in a test-tube.

'in vivo': Describing biological phenomena that occur or are observed occurring within the bodies of living organisms.

Inulin: A carbohydrate filtered from the bloodstream by the kidneys.

Isoflavone: Equal, similar, indicating isomeric compound(s) composed of equal parts within a flavone, e.g. in soy.

Isomers: Any of two or more substances whose molecules have the same atoms in different arrangements.

'K':

Keratin: A fibrous protein that forms the body's horny tissues, e.g. fingernails; also found in the skin and hair.

'L':

Lactone: Intramolecular esters of hydroxycarbonylic acids found in fragrances, e.g. peaches have more than one, and shiraz and pinot wines have a 'whiskey lactone'.

Lactose: A sugar, consisting of one molecule of glucose and one of galactose, found only in milk. Inability to absorb lactose is called lactose intolerance.

LDL (Low-Density Lipoprotein): A type of blood fat that carries cholesterol deposit in the bloodstream and in excess leads to a cholesterol build-up in the arteries.

Lecithin: One of a group of phospholipids important to cell membranes which are involved in the metabolism of fat by the liver, e.g. a nutrient occurring in animal and vegetable cells and found in unrefined 'fixed' oils.

Leucocyte (White blood cell): Any blood cell that contains a nucleus; white blood corpuscles, amoeboid cells, involved in protecting the body against foreign substances and in antibody production.

Limbic system (of the brain): A complex system of nerve pathways and networks in the brain, that is involved in the expression of instinct and mood in activities of the endocrine and motor systems of the body. Often referred to as the 'old brain ' due to its fundamental connections with self-preservation of the species, e.g. 'fight and flight'.

Linoleic acid: A plant-derived essential unsaturated fatty acid necessary to growth, which needs be included in the diet as the other two essential unsaturated fatty acids (linolenic and arachidonic acids) can be synthesised from it in the body.

Lipid: One of a group of water-insoluble important dietary constituents, giving high energy value and associated with certain vitamins and essential fatty acids.

Lipoic acid: A sulphur-containing compound that functions in carbohydrate metabolism.

Liposome: An artificial 'sac' or membrane made in the laboratory that resembles a cell membrane.

Lutein: The yellow pigment of the corpus luteum of the ovary.

Lycopene: The red carotenoid pigment of ripe tomatoes that lessens damage caused by free radicals.

Lymphatic system (of the body): A network of vessels that conveys electrolytes, water and proteins etc. in the form of lymph from the tissue fluids to the bloodstream.

Lysine: An essential amino acid.

'M':

MAOI (MAO Inhibitor): A drug that prevents the activity of the enzyme MAO (monoamine oxidase) in brain tissue and therefore affects mood. MAOIs are used as antidepressants.

Materia Medica: The repertoire of materials used in medicine, e.g. herbs used by herbalists.

Melanoma: A highly malignant tumour of melanin-forming cells, the melanocytes usually occurring in the skin as cancer, excessive sunlight being a contributory factor. It may also occur in the eye and the mucous membranes.

Melatonin: A natural hormone that is secreted during the hours of darkness by the pineal gland in the brain involved in the control of the body's circadian day/night rhythm (the ability to sleep during the hours of darkness and stay awake during daylight hours).

Mono-unsaturates: Fatty acids highly resistant to oxidation and relatively stable at high temperatures. Mono-unsaturates have a slight lowering effect on cholesterol in the blood and seem to help preserve the optimum HDL:LDL ratio.

Mucilage: A substance containing gelatinous constituents that are demulcent.

Mucopolysaccharide: One of a group of complex carbohydrates functioning mainly as structural components in connective tissue, e.g. chondroitin, occurring in cartilage.

'N':

Naturopath: One who practices naturopathy (see below).

Naturopathy: A system of medicine that relies upon the use of only 'natural' substances for the treatment of disease, rather than drugs. Including herbs, food grown without artificial fertilizers and prepared without the use of preservatives or colouring material, pure water, sunlight, and fresh air, employed in an effort to rid the body of unnatural substances, which are said to be at the root of most illnesses. Hippocrates recommended fresh air, exercise, clean water and a good diet (detoxification) and the use of eclectic traditional medicines such as herbalism to treat patients.

Nitramine: A common name for an odourless, synthetic, yellow crystal-like solid that is not found naturally in the environment – under certain conditions it can exist in dust in the air. It dissolves slightly in water and other liquids. It breaks down in soils and drinking water; one of its products is piric acid. It is not classed as carcinogenic.

Nitrogen-fixing: The ability of certain micro-organisms to 'fix' nitrogen from the air producing nitrate fertilizer. Nodules formed on the roots of members of the pea flower family contain high concentrations of such symbiotic bacteria.

Non-steroidal: Referring to NSAIDs, i.e. non-steroidal anti-inflammatory drugs that are used for pain relief, particularly in rheumatic disease, e.g. aspirin, ibuprofen.

'O':

Olfaction: The sense of smell and/or process of smelling.

Omega-3: A group of polyunsaturated essential fatty acids that comes from linolenic acid and are used by the body to produce prostaglandins and leukotrienes, similar to prostaglandins in that they control functions such as blood pressure and digestion and also help regulate inflammatory disorders such as arthritis.

Omega-6: A group of polyunsaturated essential fatty acids found in vegetable oils, e.g. corn oil.

'P':

Pantothenic acid: A part of vitamin B complex and component of coenzyme A.

Pathogen: A micro-organism, e.g. bacterium, which parasitises an animal or plant or human and produces disease.

Peristalsis: An involuntary wave-like movement that progresses along some of the hollow circular tubes of the body with longitudinal muscles, e.g. intestines.

Pharmacopoeia: A book, especially one published officially, containing a list of drugs with directions for their use.

Phenols: A group of aromatic compounds, antioxidants found in e.g. virgin olive oil and wines.

Pheromone: A chemical messenger secreted by an animal (usually associated with sexual arousal) that signals from one individual to another an internal physiological change or a change in behaviour.

Photoprotective: Protects against light, e.g. sunlight.

Phyto- (phyt-): Prefix denoting plants; of plant origin.

Pineal gland (Epiphysis): The pineal body or gland is a pea-sized mass of tissue attached by a stalk to the posterior wall of the third ventricle of the brain, deep between the cerebral hemispheres.

Pituitary gland (Hypophysis): The master endocrine gland that is attached beneath the hypothalamus in a bony cavity at the base of the skull.

Plaque: A layer that forms on the surface of a tooth, principally at its neck, composed of bacteria in an organic matrix.

Plasma (blood plasma): The straw-coloured fluid in which the blood cells are suspended.

Platelet (thrombocyte): A tiny disc-shaped structure, present in the blood, which is involved in clotting.

Polymer: A substance formed by the linkage of a large number of smaller molecules and contains many repeated units of one or more compounds, e.g. starch and plastics.

Polyphenols: Many or multiple phenols (that may affect many parts).

Polysaccharide: A carbohydrate formed from many monosaccharides joined together in long linear or branched chains. They store energy, e.g. glycogen in animals and humans, starch in plants.

Polyunsaturates: Fats (and oils) that reduce the level of cholesterol in the bloodstream but may also adversely affect the HDL:LDL ratio.

Procyanidin: Precursor of cyanidin, another name for pycnogenol.

Prostaglandin: One of a group of hormone-like substances present in a wide variety of tissues and body fluids, including the uterus, brain, lungs, kidney and semen.

Provitamin: A substance that is not itself a vitamin but can be converted to a vitamin in the body, e.g. beta-carotene converts to vitamin A.

Purine: A nitrogen-containing compound, e.g. adenine and guanine, which form the nucleotides of nucleic acids; uric acid is the end-product of purine metabolism.

Pycnogenol: A natural remedy derived commercially from grape seeds and the bark of the Mediterranean pine tree. It is a mixture of antioxidant molecules.

'R':

RDA (Recommended Daily Amount): Refers to medicine dosage and food medicine, i.e. sufficient intake of vitamins and minerals via the diet.

Reserpine: A drug extracted from Indian snakeroot, a plant of the Carribean, and used to lower high blood pressure, and occasionally to relieve anxiety.

Retinol: Vitamin A, a fat-soluble vitamin that occurs preformed in foods of animal origin and is formed in the body from the pigment beta-carotene. It is present in some vegetable foods and is essential for growth, vision in dim light, and the maintenance of soft mucous tissue. Sources include cabbage and carrots.

Riboflavin: Vitamin B_2, important in tissue respiration.

RNA (Ribonucleic acid): A nucleic acid occurring in the nucleus and cytoplasm of cells that is concerned with synthesis of proteins.

'S':

Saponifiable: Describing substances, usually fats, that can be converted into a soap by various processes.

Saponins: A group of vegetable soap-like glycosides found widely in plants that act as emulsifiers of oils and have complex effects in herbal remedies; some similar to steroidal hormones.

Scillarin: A stimulatory drug for the heart extracted from the bulbs of *D. Maritima*, 'white or red squill'. (Red bulbs also contain the rat poison scilliroside that is specific to kill rats.) Indian squill *D. indica* is another source of scillarin.

Serotonin : A compound widely distributed in the tissues, particularly in the blood platelets, the intestinal wall and central nervous system, from which it is released on activation. It is thought to play a role in inflammation similar to that of histamine, and also acts as a neurotransmitter, especially concerning the sleep process.

Serum (blood serum): The fluid that separates from clotted blood or blood plasma that is allowed to stand. It is essentially similar in composition to plasma, but lacks fibrinogen and other substances that are used in the coagulation of blood process.

SOD (Superoxide dismutase): SOD is a catalytic enzyme present in phagocytic cells – phagocytes are cells able to engulf and digest bacteria, protozoa, cells and cell debris, and other small particles – and is important to the immune system in the microbicidal activity of the cells.

Spasmolytic: A drug that relieves spasm of smooth muscle, e.g. paper-vine derived from the food medicine papaya.

Squalene: An unsaturated hydrocarbon (terepene) synthesised in the body, from which cholesterol is derived.

Statins: Lipid-lowering drugs employed for cholesterol and triglyceride fats in the blood when dietary measures have failed to control hyperlipidaemia.

Steroids: Corticosteroid drugs, often referred to simply as steroids. Naturally occurring steroids include the male and female sex hormones androgens and oestrogens. Release of these hormones is governed by the pituitary gland.

Sterol: The most important sterols are cholesterol, and ergosterol, a plant sterol that when irradiated with ultraviolet light is converted to ergocalciferol, i.e. vitamin D_2, which is necessary to the formation and maintenance of bones.

Symbiosis: An intimate and obligatory association between two different species of organism, in which there is mutual aid and benefit.

Synovial (fluid): A lubricating fluid secreted by the synovial membrane, the sac enclosing a freely movable joint.

'T':

Tannins: Astringent, sometimes slightly bitter, often antiseptic active plant constituents which precipitate proteins, e.g. tea *Camellia sinensis* syn. *Thea sinensis*, and may be used to check bleeding and discharges, e.g. *Potentilla erecta.*

Thiamine: Vitamin B_1, a coenzyme responsible for the workings of various enzymes in the body. Sources include cereals, yeast, beans, meat, potatoes and nuts.

Thiazide (diuretica): Thiazide and related compounds act on the kidneys to promote salt and water excretion.

Tocopherol: Vitamin E, involved in reproduction, the absence of which leads to sterility in both sexes. Currently often associated with cosmetics, skin condition and healing.

Triglyceride: The term applied to a fatty acid of glycerol and the basic structure of all oils and fats. It is also a fatty component in the blood related to heart disease.

'U':

Unsaturate: Fatty acids all have a long hydrocarbon chain; some of them contain double bonds and are said to be unsaturated. e.g. oleic acid found in grapeseed, olive, rose hip, safflower and sunflower oils.

Suggested Further Reading
Some Guiding Lights

Angier, Natalie: *Woman: An Intimate Geography*, Virago, 1999

Bellamy, David and Pfister, Andrea: *World Medicine*, Blackwell, 1992

Crawford, Michael and Marsh, David: *The Driving Force*, Mandarin, 1989.

Griggs, Barbara: *Green Pharmacy*, Hale, 1981

Hardin, Garrett: *Biology: Its Principles and Implications*, 1952

Houwink, R: *Sizing up Science*, John Murray, 1975

Pharmaceutical Society, The: *British Pharmaceutical Codex*, 1907

Strasburger, E: *Strasburger's Textbook of Botany*, Macmillan, 1930

Taylor, Rattray. G: *Sex in History*, Thames and Hudson, 1953

Thompson, D'Arcy. W: *On Growth and Form*, Macmillan, 1944

Vaughan, J. G. and Geissler, C. A: *The New Oxford Book of Food Plants*, Oxford, 1997